Panic on a Plate

How Society Developed an Eating Disorder

Rob Lyons

SOCIETAS

essays in political
& cultural criticism

imprint-academic.com

Published in the UK by Societas
Imprint Academic, PO Box 200, Exeter EX5 5YX, UK

Published in the USA by Societas
Imprint Academic, Philosophy Documentation Center
PO Box 7147, Charlottesville, VA 22906-7147, USA

ISBN 9781845402167

A CIP catalogue record for this book is available from the
British Library and US Library of Congress

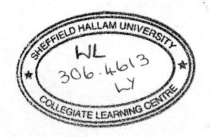

Contents

Acknowledgements

This book is an expansion of many ideas and arguments that I have discussed on *spiked* (www.spiked-online.com) and I'd like to thank everyone who has worked there for providing me with the opportunity to write and for the innumerable stimulating conversations that have helped to shape my view of the world. In particular, my former *spiked* colleague Jennie Bristow helped enormously in the process of getting these ideas down on paper. Thanks also to Michael Fitzpatrick, Tony Gilland and Jason Smith for useful comments on draft versions of the book.

Thanks also to Claire Fox, director of the Institute of Ideas, for providing me with the push to get this book started, and to Julian Hunt, formerly of the Food and Drink Federation, for providing eye-opening insights into the world of food policy and politics.

Most of all, thanks to Justine Brian for introducing me to posh nosh, debating ideas about food and simply being good company over many a good meal.

If the ideas in these pages are a feast, it is the product of many people's efforts. If what follows is a dog's dinner, blame me.

Rob Lyons
May 2011

Chapter One

Introduction

Until comparatively recently, there was only one question that the majority of people needed to ask in relation to food: how will we get enough? Most of the world's population, for most of human history, has lived in a constant struggle to obtain enough food to survive and thrive.

As Tom Standage engagingly notes in his book *An Edible History of Humanity*, the attempt to obtain food, and the way in which surplus food is used, is a major driving force of history. Civilisation is based upon the switch from hunter-gathering to settled agriculture. When farming started to produce a surplus, the monopolisation of that surplus was the basis for the creation of a ruling class in society. Food shortages have been a major factor in the outcome of wars and helped to bring down the Soviet bloc.

There are still many people—at least one billion according to the United Nations Food and Agriculture Organisation (FAO)—for whom the struggle to eat is a constant battle. It is estimated that eight million people per year die of hunger or related diseases. But for almost everyone living in developed countries and for a growing proportion of the population in developing countries, the problem of food has ceased to be about keeping body and soul together.

According to FAO statistics for 2007, for each person in the world there was food to provide an average of 2,768 calories, 76 grams of protein and 78 grams of fat per day. Not all of this food is actually consumed—much of it is wasted, as we shall see—nor is it evenly distributed. For example, people in the UK had access to the equivalent of 3,426 calories per person per day while in the war-torn Democratic

Republic of Congo, the average was just 1,500 calories per person per day. Overall, the FAO estimates that 13 per cent of the world's population was undernourished in 2007, and that the absolute number of people who experience food shortages (as opposed to the proportion of the total population that is going hungry) has been rising for over a decade.

Yet the countries that seem to be fretting most about food are the ones in which the food question, as it was historically understood, has been solved. The primary concern now seems to be that we are eating too much, of the wrong kinds of food, produced in a way that is not environmentally sustainable. The topic of food has become a hook on which to hang all sorts of prejudices and panics from class snobbery to anti-capitalism. While in most cases there is some truth to the concerns expressed, very often these fears are blown out of all proportion. The argument in this book is that Western societies are now suffering from a kind of eating disorder, where food, rather than being a source of nourishment and pleasure, has come to be seen as a source of pollution and fear.

A big fat panic

Perhaps the biggest food-related concern in recent years has been the threat of an 'obesity timebomb'. In the US and the UK, the proportion of the population that is now deemed to be obese has risen sharply in the past three decades. In relation to America's expanding waistlines, the US Center for Disease Control and Prevention (CDC) notes just how rapid the change has been:

> In 1990, among states participating in the Behavioral Risk Factor Surveillance System, 10 states had a prevalence of obesity less than 10 per cent and no states had prevalence equal to or greater than 15 per cent. By 1999, no state had prevalence less than 10 per cent, 18 states had a prevalence of obesity between 20–24 per cent, and no state had prevalence equal to or greater than 25 per cent. In 2009, only one state (Colorado) and the District of Columbia had a prevalence of obesity less than 20 per cent. Thirty-three states had a prevalence equal to or greater than 25 per cent; nine of these states (Alabama, Arkansas, Kentucky, Louisiana,

Mississippi, Missouri, Oklahoma, Tennessee, and West Virginia) had a prevalence of obesity equal to or greater than 30 per cent.[1]

In *The End of Overeating*, paediatrician and former US Food and Drug Administration (FDA) commissioner David A. Kessler notes how average weights have changed. For example, for American women aged 20–29, average weight rose from 128 pounds in 1960 to 157 pounds in 2000. For women aged 40–49 years, the change was from 142 pounds in 1960 to 169 pounds in 2000. However, he also notes how the averages hide a very dramatic divergence between the majority of the population, whose weight has increased moderately, and a minority which seems to have a strong predisposition to gain weight.[2]

In the UK the statistics are less dramatic, but there has been, until very recently, a trend towards rising rates of obesity. In 1980, less than 10 per cent of the UK population was considered to be obese. By 2008, 24 per cent of women and 25 per cent of men fell into the obese category. Recent official statistics suggest that Britain's weight gain has plateaued, at least for now.[3] The rise in obesity rates may also be levelling off in the US.[4]

Yet the UK and US are not the fattest nations on earth – other countries with smaller populations, such as Samoa, Jordan and Saudi Arabia are even heavier. Indeed, the rise of obesity is a worldwide phenomenon, with substantial portions of the populations of developing countries deemed to be overweight, particularly those living in cities.

Does the growth of the human girth matter? The official line is 'yes – and Something Must Be Done'. Obesity has been associated in numerous studies with a variety of

---

[1] CDC 'Obesity Trends Among U.S. Adults Between 1985 and 2009' accessed at http://1.usa.gov/ed72IF
[2] Kessler, D. 2009, *The End of Overeating: Taking Control of Our Insatiable Appetites*, Penguin
[3] Department of Health, *Health Survey for England – 2009*: Adult trend tables
[4] Flegal, K. *et al.*, 2010, Prevalence and Trends in Obesity Among US Adults, 1999–2008, *Journal of the American Medical Association*, 303(3):235–241

chronic conditions, particularly heart disease, cancer and type-2 diabetes. If we do not tackle the problem of obesity, we are warned, millions will die and many more will suffer years of ill-health. In 2004, the US secretary of health Tommy Thompson declared that 400,000 Americans were dying every year because of their weight. The British celebrity chef and food campaigner, Jamie Oliver, has warned that children will die at a younger age than their parents if eating habits don't change. Governments around the world have launched all manner of campaigns to try to get their citizens to cut the calories and do more exercise in a bid to reverse the rise in obesity. Yet, as I examine in chapter 4, it is questionable whether the simple equation 'obesity = disease' is actually true.

Junk culture

The current obsession with the nation's diet is not restricted to how much we eat, but also includes attempts to micromanage what we eat. A survey for the UK Food Standards Agency published in February 2010 showed that only 35 per cent of adults — and just 15 per cent of teenagers — consumed the recommended five portions of fruit and vegetables per day.[5] Intakes of saturated fats and sugar remained above the government's 'target levels', while consumption of oily fish and dietary fibre was considered too low.

All sorts of fantastic claims are made about the importance of eating these recommended foods, usually based on limited research, to the point where nobody raises an eyebrow at the notion of national governments setting targets for their citizens' fish consumption. Our salad-dodging ways apparently mean that we may be missing out on important nutrients, and not just the obvious ones like protein, vitamins and minerals. Flavonoids and antioxidants, omega-3 fatty acids and numerous other micro-nutrients have had grand claims made about their health-preserving

---

[5]   Decade of spending on health messages 'has had little effect', *Independent*, 10 February 2010

powers in recent years, from preventing heart attacks to improving learning.

Indeed, poor diet has been claimed to be the root of anti-social behaviour in and out of the classroom. In 2008, John Stein, professor of physiology at Oxford University, told *The Times*:

> We see on TV every day somebody who has been stabbed or shot. That is often a consequence of people not being able to control their anger, and being unable to focus their attention on the consequences of their actions. I think this can be caused by a slight impairment of the prefrontal cortex — the part of the brain that is most sensitive to lack of key nutrients.[6]

This reductionist thinking also played a part in celebrity chef Jamie Oliver's campaigning TV series *Jamie's School Dinners*, which was based on the premise that children who ate better, particularly by consuming slowly digested meals rather than quick calories from sugary 'junk' food, would concentrate better in class and would be less likely to misbehave. This argument appeared to gain support from a study in the *Journal of Health Economics* in April 2011, which found that pupils in the schools that had introduced the new 'healthier' meals had seen small improvements in the number of pupils achieving the higher standard for English and Science and a decline in absences. But to what extent this small effect can really be put down to the chemical composition of the food is unclear.[7]

The changing constitution of our diets is also being blamed for the rise in obesity. Many writers, including David A. Kessler, argue that a lot of people are now actually addicted to the food they eat. Kessler describes a veteran war correspondent ('Andrew'), and his battle with junk-food temptation:

> The food industry has been remarkably successful at designing foods to capture the attention of people like him. Food manufacturers, food designers, and restaurant own-

[6] Better diet could stop criminals from getting a taste of porridge, *The Times*, 29 January 2008

[7] Belot, M., James, J. (2011) Healthy school meals and educational outcomes, *Journal of Health Economics*

ers may not fully understand the science behind the appeal
of their foods, but they know that sugar, fat and salt sell. As
surely as if he were wearing a bull's-eye on his chest,
Andrew is one of the industry's targets.

Kessler asserts that malevolent fast-food industry execu-
tives have got us all fat by cynically targeting our 'reward
centres', caring little for the health of their customers. Many
of these customers are helpless, Kessler argues, in the face of
a packet of M&M's, a tub of ice cream or a box of fried
chicken.

Malevolent industry is a long-running theme addressed
by numerous other writers, including American authors
Eric Schlosser (*Fast Food Nation*) and Michael Pollan (*The
Omnivore's Dilemma*), and British writers like Joanna
Blythman (*Bad Food Britain*) and Felicity Lawrence (*Eat Your
Heart Out*). We are the poor saps who cannot resist the
mixture of marketing and biochemistry employed by the
fast-food chains and major supermarkets. Only by breaking
free from the iron grip of Big Food, goes the argument,
can we restore a previous Golden Age of health and self-
reliance.

Ethical eating

All of this places an impossible moral burden upon food,
particularly well illustrated by TV campaigns around
animal welfare brought to us both by Jamie Oliver and his
fellow celebrity chef, Hugh Fearnley-Whittingstall. Among
other things, these campaigning shows have suggested that
cheap chicken is fattier than the free-range equivalent
(apparently, that's bad for us), and that the cramped and
ever-so short lives of broiler chickens should be a source of
shame to us all. If only on moral grounds, we should reject
such cut-price meat in favour of more expensive, but more
'ethical' alternatives.

'Ethical living' is also at the heart of concerns about how
our eating habits affect the environment. Is industrialised
agriculture, which has been the basis of the ready availability of food since the Second World War in developed countries, actually destroying the planet—and if so, what should

we do about it? Many campaigners believe that artificial fertilisers, derived from atmospheric nitrogen by using large
quantities of natural gas, are contributing to global warming, as is the transportation of food for thousands of miles
around the world. Is it ethical, they ask, to buy green beans
from Kenya or lamb from New Zealand when transporting
such foods involves substantial greenhouse-gas emissions?

This ethical outlook suggests the rejection of our current
agricultural system in favour of one based on more
traditional methods — like organic fertilisers and natural
pesticides — and for a far higher proportion of our food to be
grown locally. Indeed, some groups — so called 'locavores' —
have committed themselves to only eating food that is
seasonal and produced within a short distance of where
they live. One example is provided by the followers of the
'Fife Diet', who endeavour to eat only food produced within
100 miles of their homes in east Scotland.

A related idea is that we should cut down, or even give
up, our consumption of meat. A widely quoted statistic is
that 18 per cent of global greenhouse gas emissions are the
product of meat production — far more than even those produced by cars, planes and other forms of transportation.
The idea of going veggie for the planet has been promoted
by a range of high-profile figures, from the head of the Intergovernmental Panel on Climate Change (IPCC), Rajendra
Pachauri, to former Beatle Sir Paul McCartney.

Food as a slice of modern life

The argument of this book is that while there is an element
of truth to many of these concerns, the panics associated
with food are out of all proportion with reality. In fact, I
would argue that most of the concerns about food have very
little to do with food itself but reflect the way that we understand society more generally. In particular, a number of
themes emerge from our multifarious worries about food.

Firstly, there is a diminished sense of humanity's capabil-
ities and, by implication, an exaggerated sense of our vulnerability. For example, the fact that such a large proportion

of the world's population can now be fed is a remarkable achievement. Far from a growing population leaving many more people hungry, as a variety of Malthus-inspired doomsayers suggested in the 1960s, the number of calories available per head rose from 2,254 in 1961 to 2,768 in 2007.

Yet popular discussion focuses not on the fact that we have done this before, but on the assumption that increasing food production to such an extent again must be impossible. As my colleague at *spiked*, Brendan O'Neill, has pointed out, the idea of that there are 'too many people' has gone from taboo to common sense in just a few years.[8]

Or take a look at the issue of obesity. Rather than taking a step back and understanding that over-nutrition is a far better problem to have than under-nutrition, mainstream commentary frets about a terrifying toll in the future of weight-related illness and death. This prospect has been, to use fast-food parlance, super-sized. The overwhelming majority of obese people — who are only really fat in the eyes of medical statisticians, not by the standards of their friends and family — can look forward to a life expectancy very similar to that of their more slender peers.

The issue of food addiction brings out the downbeat view of people that rests at the heart of many food panics. Never mind that we are conscious beings balancing a whole range of influences in making our eating decisions: the idea that some wicked concoction of sugar, fat and salt 'makes' us gorge ourselves equates human beings with lab rats. Suddenly, we are relieved of the responsibility of dealing with our own lives and we can blame our failings on evil corporations while fetishising foodstuffs.

Another theme that will become apparent in this book is the way that food panics have entered into the void left by the collapse of political life. Those who want to pronounce on food seem often to be the most petty, individualistic and fearful, dripping with hatred for the two great opposing poles of society: big business to the right, the working class to the left. With the workers no longer revolting and the

[8]   The 'taboo' they just can't stop talking about, *spiked*, 17 February 2010

bourgeoisie finding it hard to trumpet the wonders of the free market, other sections of society, whose voices would once have been drowned out, have come to the fore — particularly in the way food is discussed in the media.

Thus, the discussion of food — like that of a great deal in society today — is dominated by a middle-class outlook. Not middle-class in the sense of middle income, but in the sense of arising from sections of society that are constantly threatened with being squeezed out of modern life and hence react against modernity: small business people and the self-employed, like farmers and shopkeepers; the old aristocracy and the landed gentry; the remnants of the Church of England; the journalist and the celebrity chef.

The result is a discussion about food that is quick to blame big corporations for wrecking the quaint world of small producers and retailers and which simultaneously looks down on the masses for their 'tacky', greedy eating habits. In this snobbish way of looking at food, what we eat is a lifestyle choice, a way of playing with identity, of making a difference to 'the planet'... it's anything but a way of providing fuel to live. All this handwringing about food has also provided a way for governments to connect with the populace, through telling us how and what to eat.

What I want to offer is a humane and rational view of how we could approach food. Things have never been this good, let us relax and enjoy our good fortune while striving both to make things even better here and to make sure that everyone in the world can take a seat at the feast.

This panic on our plates is robbing us of the pleasure of food. Rather than revelling in the cornucopia that society now provides, we fret about waistline inches and food miles. Parents are left to wonder if every little treat is really a poison. Every mouthful becomes something to be feared, even just a little, rather than fully enjoyed. A Frenchman once said that the English had 200 religions, but only one sauce. Well, religion ain't what it used to be and the one sauce is now a rather bitter one: guilt. It's time we tackled our eating disorder.

Chapter Two

How has our food changed?

One of the prejudices of the food debate today is that there was a Golden Age in which everyone ate well, with lots of locally produced meat, fruit and vegetables, lovingly prepared at home. All this could be purchased from the friendly, local greengrocer, butcher and baker, who would be ready with a smile and a little local gossip. Eating out was rare and convenience food non-existent.

This idyll is presented in sharp contrast to a modern way of eating, built on ready meals, fast food and 'junk'. Our children allegedly grow up on sweets and crisps, and wouldn't recognise a real vegetable if it bit them. If only we could return to those home-cooked meals of yore, goes the misty-eyed argument, then all of our problems of obesity and ill-health would disappear.

But both sides of this image are exaggerated. The working classes in Britain did not eat well until comparatively recently. Food was expensive relative to many people's incomes and what they could afford was often monotonous and dull. It is only with rising living standards, falling food prices and the appearance of the much-maligned supermarket that a wide range of foods was available at affordable prices to the majority. Moreover, the 'home-grown' past was built on the hard labour of women, who stayed at home to raise families and were able to devote long periods of time to buying food and cooking it.

A high-profile version of this idea is promoted by the American academic and food writer, Michael Pollan, in his bestselling *In Defence of Food*. Pollan presents us with some handy food rules, summed up in the seven-word motto: 'Eat food. Not too much. Mostly plants.' And what does Pollan mean by food? 'Don't eat anything your great-great-grandmother wouldn't recognize as food.' As a note of explanation, he adds: 'Sorry, but at this point Moms are as confused as the rest of us, which is why we have to go back a couple of generations, to a time before the advent of modern food products.'[1]

It seems a little strange that we should be fretting about our eating habits when cookery books and shows are so ubiquitous. We are surrounded by Jamie Oliver, Delia Smith, Nigel Slater, Nigella Lawson, Gordon Ramsay, Hugh Fearnley-Whittingstall, Sophie Dahl, the Hairy Bikers, Rick Stein and many more. Jamie Oliver has become a one-man food industry. His most recent book, *Jamie's 30-Minute Meals*, is the fastest selling non-fiction book in UK publishing history: only JK Rowling's Harry Potter books have sold faster. BBC1 television gives over a great chunk of its Saturday mornings to Saturday Kitchen, while food-related shows like *Masterchef* (in no less than three different formats), *Hell's Kitchen*, *Ready Steady Cook*, *The Great British Bake-Off*, *The Great British Menu* and many more would suggest that we are a nation in love with food and cooking.

Others have called our modern obsession with cookery 'food porn': an apt description of an interest in food that is all about watching and not about doing. British food writer Joanna Blythman is, to a degree, right to be sceptical of the idea that the nation's food culture has undergone a renaissance:

> Nowadays, Britain so desperately wants to be seen as a fully functioning, participatory food culture that it feeds this delusion by selectively ignoring the gaping discrepancies that don't fit. Most glaringly, there's our growing incompetence in the domestic kitchen and our increasing

[1] *Unhappy Meals*, by Michael Pollan,
http://michaelpollan.com/articles-archive/unhappy-meals

> reluctance to cook—surely the most telling indicator of a
> nation's culinary health? How many people do you know
> who still consider it a priority to cook from scratch a sim-
> ple, home-made meal most days of the week?[2]

As it happens, Blythman may be overly pessimistic. A
survey on British eating habits conducted for the Food
Standards Agency reported in March 2011 that 'almost
three-fifths (57 per cent) said they cooked or prepared food
for themselves every day, and 37 per cent did so for others'.
A majority of respondents agreed with the statements 'I
enjoy cooking and preparing food' (68 per cent), and 'I enjoy
making new things to eat' (65 per cent). The majority (65 per
cent) disagreed with the statement 'For me, food is just fuel
to live'. Overall, 40 per cent agreed with 'Cooking is like a
hobby for me'.

Jamie Oliver also laments the demise of 'real food', and
illustrates this by showing how many children cannot
recognise common vegetables. In his US television series
Jamie Oliver's Food Revolution, Oliver visits a class of
six-year-olds in West Virginia and asks them to identify a
variety of vegetables. He's shocked to find that the children
failed the task. (Though he really shouldn't be—he performed precisely the same demonstration in his UK series
Jamie's School Dinners a few years earlier.) They knew what
tomato ketchup was, but didn't recognise tomatoes. They
thought an eggplant might be a pear and guessed that a beet
was celery. This seems dramatic, but what did Oliver's
stunt actually prove? Quite apart from the fact that such
young children don't know much about anything at all, one
blogger pointed out that it was as much an indication that
the children didn't read. After all, the alphabet is often illustrated with vegetables for the letters—C is for Carrot, and so
on. And if children don't know how to name whole vegetables, it does not necessarily mean that they don't, or won't,
eat them.

[2]   Can't cook, won't cook, by Joanna Blythman, *Observer Food Monthly*,
28 May 2006

Council-house cuisine

So, if we accept for a moment that we don't have a great food culture now, did we have one in the past? I would argue that urban Britain had a limited range of food in the past and, if we ate home-cooked food, it was as much out of necessity as choice. I was born in the late 1960s and grew up in a council house in Birmingham. My widowed mother raised the family on welfare benefits and her part-time job as a school dinner lady (Jamie would approve). When we got home, my mother would cook every night, except on the rare occasions when I'd be sent off to buy fish and chips. My mother's cooking was rarely sophisticated fare: meat and two veg, with cottage pie or stew for variety, and the occasional excursion into fancy foreign stuff like spaghetti. Even living in the multicultural, inner-city district of Sparkbrook (home to the 'Balti Triangle' of cut-price, family-run Indian restaurants), my first taste of curry came from a reconstituted packet mix made by a company called Vesta.

So, while we had plenty of home-cooked food, our horizons were pretty narrow. Vegetables were potatoes, cabbage, peas, carrots and onions. Salad was lettuce, tomatoes and cucumber with beetroot from a jar. Sweetcorn arrived like some fluorescent exotica when I was in my teens. At university, I went to visit a middle-class friend who lived in the relatively well-to-do town of Cheltenham. She decided to cook and I was intrigued to see that she was frying cucumber, something I'd never come across before. 'They're not cucumbers!', she exclaimed. 'They're courgettes!' Guffaws all round, at my expense.

I had managed to remain completely ignorant of a common vegetable till the age of 19, despite the fact that I grew up in a household where home-cooked meals were the order of the day. All it proved was that my mother was fairly conservative and how much we needed a decent supermarket nearby.

A bite-sized history of eating

My comparatively limited food horizons were still a major step forward from the eating habits of the working classes in the past. The middle classes have always managed to eat well. Back in the nineteenth century, a reasonably well-off family would have eaten meals that were a little quaint to our eyes but were varied and interesting. But the working class survived on meagre rations, mostly of bread and potatoes. In a study published in 1970 of 151 individual family budgets from investigations undertaken between 1887 and 1901, D.J. Oddy found a weekly average diet per head of 6.7 pounds of bread, 1.6 pounds of potatoes, 14 ounces of sugar, 2.8 ounces of cereals, 4.9 ounces of fat, 1.4 pounds of meat and 1.4 pints of milk. These averages hide the degree to which women would have made do with even less to ensure that the breadwinners could eat better. In these budgets, women ate little more than half the calories and less than half the protein of men.[3]

The Victorian conservative reformer and researcher, Charles Booth, noted that for regularly employed unskilled workers, as opposed to the abjectly poor, there was generally enough to eat:

> For dinner, meat and vegetables are demanded every day. Bacon, eggs and fish find their place at other times. Puddings and tarts are not uncommon and bread ceases to be the staff of life. Skill in cookery becomes very important and, though capable of much improvement, it is on the whole not amiss. In this class, no one goes short of food.[4]

This was no longer the tedious diet of bread that the truly poor suffered, but it was hardly a rich culinary tapestry either.

One thing of note in Oddy's article is that the inclination of the government to lecture the poor on their eating habits is nothing new. Oddy quotes the Inter-Departmental Commission on Physical Deterioration from 1904: 'It is no doubt the case that with greater knowledge, the poor might live

---

[3]   Oddy, D.J. (1970) 'Working-class Diets in Late Nineteenth-Century Britain', *The Economic History Review*

[4]   Quoted in Oddy (1970), op cit

more cheaply than they do, but with all classes the tendency is to spend as little as possible on food.' The problem was a desire to make food palatable when more calories and protein could have been obtained simply from eating more of the staple foods. The Committee blamed this on a 'desire for some sort of sensation, comparable to the... dietary of pickles and vinegar'.

In *The Road to Wigan Pier*, George Orwell describes how he was confronted by this tendency for the well-off to lecture the poor. During his travels, Orwell encountered a communist who was incensed by the attempts of the upper classes to 'teach the unemployed more about food values': 'Parties of society dames now have the cheek to walk into East End houses and give shopping lessons to the wives of the unemployed...' Now they would have shows on Channel 4.

The results from Oddy's work are confirmed by Maud Pember Reeves's 1914 book *Round About a Pound a Week*, based on survey work undertaken in the London borough of Lambeth amongst families with regular work:

> Without doubt, the chief article of diet in a 20-shilling budget is bread. A long way after bread come potatoes, meat, and fish. Bread is bought from one of the abundance of bakers in the neighbourhood, and is not as a rule very different in price and quality from bread in other parts of London. Meat is generally bargained for on street stalls on Saturday night or even Sunday morning. It may be cheaper than meat purchased in the West End, but is certainly worse in original quality as well as less fresh and less clean in condition. Potatoes are generally two pounds for a penny, unless they are 'new' potatoes.[5]

Even if there had been a wide variety of foods available, cooking them would have been tricky, as Reeves notes:

> Another difficulty which dogs the path of the Lambeth housekeeper is, either that there is no oven or only a gas oven which requires a good deal of gas, or that the stove oven needs much fuel to heat it. Once a week, for the Sunday dinner, the plunge is taken. Homes where there is no oven send out to the bakehouse on that occasion. The

[5]   Pember Reeves, M. (1913) *Round About A Pound Per Week*

rest of the week is managed on cold food, or the hard-worked saucepan and frying-pan are brought into play.

By 1936, the Conservative MP—and later first head of the UN Food and Agriculture Organisation—John Boyd Orr would report in Food, Health and Income that 'a diet completely adequate for health, according to modern standards, is reached at an income level above 50 per cent of the population'.[6] In other words, many people could still not afford to feed themselves and their families properly.

Boyd Orr notes some significant changes over time in the percentage of income spent on food and what it was spent on. A hundred years previously, almost half of income per head was spent on food, but this had fallen to about 30 per cent by 1934. Moreover, what could be bought for that proportion of wages had changed: the amount of tea per head per week went from half an ounce to three ounces; sugar consumption rose five-fold. On the other hand, Boyd Orr found that milk consumption was no higher while consumption of bread and flour had been 80 per cent higher in 1836 than in 1934.

Better comparative figures were available to Boyd Orr from the periods 1909–13 and 1924–28. Consumption per head of many foods rose between the earliest of these periods and the latest: fruit (up 88 per cent); vegetables (up 164 per cent); butter (up 57 per cent); cheese (up 43 per cent). However, for meat and potatoes, consumption barely changed while wheat flour consumption fell a little. In terms of the nutrient content of people's diets, there was a small increase in animal protein, a bigger rise in fat consumption and a slight fall in carbohydrates—which, added together, produced a small increase in overall calories consumed.

The book's analysis of diets by income group is revealing. Boyd Orr found that the rich ate more meat, milk, eggs, cheese, fruit and vegetables than the poor. Some of Boyd Orr's data suggest that the poor made up for this by eating

---

[6]   Boyd Orr, J. (1936) *Food, Health & Income: Report on a Survey of Adequacy of Diet in Relation to Income*

more bread and potatoes, but the national estimates he provides suggest that all social classes ate much the same amount of these cheap staples. The key factors in changing this situation were rising wages and the falling cost of some foods, driven by the industrialisation of agriculture. Particularly after the Second World War, food became much more plentiful. Moreover, the postwar period saw a complete change in the way food was prepared. Not only did families have kitchens and cookers, but items like refrigerators and freezers became progressively more common, allowing the storage of food in a way previously not possible.

As a result of rising living standards, the proportion of household budgets spent on food has fallen from 30 per cent in John Boyd Orr's report in 1936, to 21 per cent in 1971, to a mere nine per cent by 2007.

The joy of convenience

What we eat may have changed, but how we shop for, store and prepare it has changed, too. In terms of shopping, the major change has been the rise of the supermarket and the demise of the daily shop. In her history of the wartime Ministry of Food, Jane Fearnley-Whittingstall notes how 'most women dreaded the drudgery of wartime shopping':

> It's difficult to imagine just how different buying food was in the 1930s and 1940s. Instead of stocking up weekly at the supermarket, women walked or cycled to their local high street to call at the butcher, the baker, the grocer, the fishmonger and the greengrocer. They invariably had to queue for anything up to an hour, come rain or shine, snow or sleet. And shopping was almost a daily occurrence; without fridges or freezers, perishable food that might 'go off' had to be bought in small quantities. [7]

The supermarket, in combination with refrigeration and the motor car, not only made shopping more convenient, it also greatly increased the range of foods we could obtain. A friend of mine who grew up in London in the 1970s recalls the range of cheeses available in her local shop: yellow or

---

[7]   Fearnley-Whittingstall, J. (2010) *Ministry of Food: Thrifty Wartime Ways to Feed Your Family Today*

orange. In the 1995 edition of her *Complete Cookery Course*, Delia Smith writes about what had changed since writing the first edition: 'What, 14 years ago, had to be sought out in specialised food shops is now widely available in super-markets up and down the country. Almost everyone now has access to good olive oil, fresh herbs, imported cheeses. I found myself over and over again deleting the words "or if you can't get it …".'

For those of us brought up in working-class industrial and post-industrial towns, the supermarket opened up hither-to unthinkable culinary opportunities. Of course, it wasn't all parmesan and courgettes — there were family packs of crisps and cod fish fingers, too, but for the first time, we had the choice.

Alongside the posh new ingredients came convenience. In the UK, Marks and Spencer took the lead in providing chilled ready meals, but the supermarkets weren't far behind. For housewives going to work in ever-greater num-bers, the idea of preparing something tasty with little effort was a real boon. The microwave oven made things even quicker.

As it goes, convenience was not entirely new. We can, apparently, thank America's celebration of Thanksgiving for the TV Dinner. The 'TV Dinner' was a brand of frozen ready meal invented in 1953 by C.A. Swanson, a major American food company. The story goes that the firm had massively overestimated how many turkeys it would need to meet Thanksgiving demand. How to get rid of the excess? The company realised that packaging the whole Thanksgiving meal on one, compartmentalised aluminium tray that you could pop in the oven, then tuck into in front of the television, might be popular with customers. They reckoned they would sell 5,000 in the first year. They sold 10 million. As one wag wrote in the *Christian Science Monitor* a few years ago: they came, they thawed, they conquered.

Mass production of frozen food goes back even further. The process was developed in 1923 by Clarence Birdseye. (Sadly, it seems Birdseye wasn't a ship's captain with a gnarly voice and a crew of child pirates who ate fish fingers all the time, as depicted in British TV adverts for decades, but an American inventor.) We can go back still further to the invention of canning, in the early nineteenth century.

Another myth is the idea that we have now become a takeaway culture when in the past we cooked at home. As noted above, Maud Pember Reeves found inner-city Londoners had very limited cooking facilities, so preparing hot food at home was tricky. But in any event, Britain has had its own, homegrown fast-food joints for well over a century. As John K. Walton notes in his history of fish and chip shops, these takeaways 'came to be almost ubiquitous in industrial Britain by the early twentieth century, after a period of accelerating growth in shop numbers and colonisation of new territories from the late 1870s and early 1880s'. Nor were these the preserve of the few. Walton writes that 'working-class families in industrial areas used the fish and chip shop three or four times a week'.

Walton describes a moralistic debate about the dangers of the chippy, which echoes the modern concerns about fast food:

> There was also a contemporary debate over fish and chips and working-class living standards. Critics alleged that fish and chips was indigestible, expensive and unwhole-some. It was seen as a route to, or an aspect of, the 'second-ary poverty' which arose from the incompetent or immoral misapplication of resources that would otherwise have been sufficient to sustain an adequate standard of living. It was presented as part of a pathology of culinary ignorance and the failure to use cheap ingredients to their best advan-tage. Above all, perhaps, it was seen as an easy way of avoiding the full burden of household responsibilities.[8]

In his book *From Plain Fare to Fusion Food: British Diet from the 1890s to the 1990s*, Oddy notes that in Blackpool, 'a seaside town of some 50,000 residents when not swollen by summer visitors, the list of places supplying food in 1906 included 182 sweet-shops, 79 fish, chip and tripe shops, and 58 res-taurants'. Burgers came to Britain in 1953, when Wimpy set up hamburger counters in Lyons tea rooms. (Sadly, the

---

[8] Walton, J.K. (1994) *Fish and Chips and the British Working Class, 1870–1940*

Lyons of tea room fame was no relation to me: the company was, however, co-founded by Nigella Lawson's great-great-grandfather.) The first motorway service stations were opened by Forte in 1960 at Newport Pagnall and Watford Gap on the M1. Pizza Hut arrived in 1973, two years ahead of McDonald's.

While the degree to which we eat outside the home may have increased, the use of takeaways and cafés is not novel by any means. Nor is convenience entirely new, though it is true that fewer meals are prepared from scratch at home than ever before. However, this is not because we've been duped into doing this by mega-corporations—it is because we find living this way to be convenient.

One consequence of the fact that more of our food is prepared by others is that there is a greater space opened up for us to be fearful about food. If food is something we consume but don't prepare, then we have to have faith that those who are cooking that takeaway or manufacturing that ready meal are doing so to a high standard. It is this gap between creator and consumer that helps to increase the possibility for food panics.

Chapter Three

The myth of junk food

Is there such a thing as 'real' food and 'junk' food? One of the symptoms of our societal eating disorder is to categorise food into good and bad. That might make some sense when it comes to aesthetics—'Does it taste good?'—but such terms are generally used in quite a different way.

Yet what is categorised as 'junk' is often more nutritious than that which is regarded as wholesome. Underpinning much of the discussion of 'real' food and 'junk' food is a snobbery towards those who enjoy, or rely upon, processed food and an exaggerated suspicion of all things corporate. As we saw in the last chapter, that snobbery is not new.

The term 'junk food' is generally believed to have been coined in 1972 by Michael Jacobson of the US Center for Science in the Public Interest (CSPI), a consumer advocacy group that specialises in food issues. The *Oxford English Dictionary* defines junk food as 'pre-prepared or packaged food that has low nutritional value'. Junk food is, we are told, at best bad for our waistlines and, at worst, poison for our kids.

Junk is big business. Datamonitor put the global savoury snacks market alone at $46 billion in 2005, while worldwide confectionery sales in 2008 amounted to $127 billion. Breakfast cereals — with worldwide sales of $24.5 billion in 2008 — are heavily advertised with claims about being healthy. Yet such products are often simply cheap cereals like maize heavily laden with salt and sugar, with a few added vitamins to boost their claims to be nutritious. Are we being sold poor-quality food dressed up by misleading promotion to appear to be something more exciting than it is? In *The End of Food*, Paul Roberts points out:

Food processors have become so adept at adding value that
by the end of the process, the initial cost of the grain or
other raw materials is only a tiny fraction of the retail price;
of the $3.50 you pay for a 12-ounce box of cereal at the
supermarket, less than 25 cents represents the cost of the
grain itself.

While this is a little disingenuous, given how many other
costs in terms of labour, transport and a profit for the store
are included in that retail price, it also shows that branding
can go a long way in bumping up the price of products
based on cheap ingredients.

Perhaps even more concerning, for campaigners and
health officials, is the proliferation of fast-food joints
around the world: McDonald's, Burger King, Wendy's,
Pizza Hut, KFC, plus many other chains and one-off restaurants and takeaways have proliferated in recent decades.
According to the business information company
IBISWorld, there were 303,000 'limited service' restaurants
in the US in 2009, employing nearly four million people and
raking in $178 billion in revenues. McDonald's alone has
over 31,000 restaurants in 119 countries.

If health officials and foodies are to be believed, this
explosion of junk means we are on the road to hell. In July
2010, for example, the leaders of two royal colleges of medicine in the UK demanded a crackdown on junk food. Professor Dinesh Bhugra, president of the Royal College of
Psychiatrists, told the *Guardian*:

> Some types of processed foods are harmful to the physical,
> and consequently mental, health of individuals. There
> ought to be serious consideration given to banning adver-
> tising of certain foods and certain processed foods and to
> levying tax on fatty, unhealthy foods, which would be
> ring-fenced for the NHS, which deals with the conse-
> quences of fatty foods.[1]

Indeed, the UK's communications regulator Ofcom has
already taken a step down this road, introducing a ban in
2008 on adverts for foods high in fat, salt and sugar during
television programmes aimed at children under the age of

[1]   Leading doctors call for urgent crackdown on junk food, *Guardian*, 11
       July 2010

16. This was despite protests from programme-makers that the lost advertising revenue could seriously affect the already hard-pressed budgets for original productions and doubts over whether such a ban would have any significant effect on eating habits.

Junk food is allegedly as addictive as heroin and cocaine — and just as deadly. Take this statement from British TV gardener and food campaigner Monty Don:

> Consumption of these foods leads to poor health and as such they are poisoning our children. They are all highly addictive; by the time children reach the kind of age where they can reasonably exercise choice, let alone be equipped to make one, they are hopelessly hooked on junk.[2]

Spot the difference

But does the idea that junk food is less nutritious than 'real' food stand up to close examination? For example, take the classic Big Mac meal from McDonald's. The sandwich contains about 500 calories, including two thin slices of ground beef and a slice of processed cheese. The accompanying fries are actually surprisingly nutritious — french fries contain substantially more vitamin C, pound-for-pound, than apples. A portion of fries contains between one quarter and one third of the daily requirements for vitamin C for an adult.

Even the ubiquitous tomato ketchup is a surprisingly healthy product — but that really shouldn't be surprising since it is essentially concentrated tomatoes with a little vinegar, salt and sugar. According to the US Department of Agriculture (USDA) food database, 25g of ketchup contains 25 calories, barely any fat and about 0.25 grams of sodium. But it also contains six per cent of an adult's recommended daily intake of vitamin C and about 4.5 per cent of vitamin A requirements.

As Stanley Feldman notes in *Panic Nation*: 'The term "junk food" is an oxymoron. Either something is a food, in

---

[2]   We are being ruled by a junk-food government, *Guardian*, 11 July 2010

which case it is not junk, or it has no nutritional value, in which case it cannot be called a food.'[3]

Another example might be the much-maligned doner kebab: minced, spiced lamb served with salad in pitta bread. It may be very greasy—the kebabs need to be made with a lot of fat to allow them to cook on the rotisserie without burning—but the doner kebab constitutes a good and nutritious meal, if a highly calorific one.

The idea that a McDonald's meal or a doner kebab is pretty good nutritionally would obviously send our health guardians into apoplectic fits. There's too much sugar, too much fat, not enough vegetables. (In the world of the food police, potatoes don't count as vegetables.) But while living relentlessly on a diet of nothing but takeaways might ultimately mean missing out on one or two nutrients—never mind being a bit tedious—it is certainly at least as nutritious as the alternatives offered up as superior.

For example, how about a nice salad? All those lovely crunchy leaves, a few tomatoes, perhaps some kind of protein like chicken or tuna? Try living on that for a few weeks and watch yourself waste away or spend all your time chomping in order to get enough calories to survive. While such a diet would be rich in many vitamins, it would simply not contain enough energy to satisfy the normal needs of an adult man or woman. Becoming stick thin, and living with a constant craving for food, might be a reasonable sacrifice for a wannabe Hollywood starlet, but it's no way for the rest of us to live.

There is a much-mythologised tale that the US government under President Reagan considered redefining tomato ketchup as a fruit/vegetable. But in terms of its nutritional content, such an idea isn't all that terrible. According to those US figures, ketchup contains three times as much vitamin C, pound for pound, as apples. One objection might be that the ketchup contains twice as much sugar, but that still means you get less sugar for each unit of vitamin C with ketchup than you do with apples. That's

---

[3]   Feldman, S., Marks, V. (2005) *Panic Nation*

right: apples, not ketchup, are the sugary, vitamin-lite option. So which one is the junk food?

The discussion about what is and what is not 'junk food' reached its nadir with the Ofcom regulation of advertising introduced in 2008. A ban on 'foods high in fat, salt and sugar' catches a lot of things that foodies would consider rather good. Cheese is roughly one third fat. Parmesan is also pretty salty. Olive oil is pure fat. Butter must be, by law, 80 per cent fat. Yet as chef-turned-author Anthony Bourdain points out in his bestseller, *Kitchen Confidential*, explaining why restaurant food tastes better than home-cooked: 'I don't care what they tell you they're putting or not putting in your food at your favourite restaurant, chances are you're eating a ton of butter. In a professional kitchen, it's almost always the first and last thing in the pan.'

Honey and raisins—usually regarded as 'good'—are practically pure sugar. Orange juice, according to the USDA, is 87 per cent water; almost all the rest is sugar.

Let's turn the tables for a moment in this junk food discussion: If a big processed-food manufacturer came up with a product called 'Orange Fun' that tasted overpoweringly of oranges but was essentially water, sugar and a little vitamin C, it would be condemned out of hand by foodies. Yet that's what orange juice is—it's just 'natural'. On the same theme, if such a manufacturer produced a milk for infants that had less protein and more fat and allergy-inducing lactose than full-fat cow's milk, there would be uproar, especially if that company tried to persuade the government to bully every mother into using it. No need to bother, the product is already widely available under the name 'breast milk'.[4]

Caviar is saltier than seawater; tinned anchovies are three times saltier than seawater. Should these foods be on the 'junk' list? Salt is an absolutely essential ingredient to enhance flavour, yet certain kinds of salty foods are considered delicacies, while others are considered junk.

---

[4]   Whole milk, USDA Nutrition Database, http://www.nal.usda.gov/ fnic/foodcomp/cgi-bin/list_nut_edit.pl; Jenness, R. (1979) The composition of human milk, *Seminars in Perinatology*, Jul;3(3):225–39

A sense of perspective is required on what is and is not a good diet. For example, consider the diets of those who live in many developing countries where junk food is unheard of and a 'staple' food really means something. There, one food may dominate people's diets, be it rice, bread, maize or cassava. Meat and vegetables are added when available, but the diet remains quite limited. Can that seriously be described as better than living off burgers, pizzas, kebabs and fried chicken?

The need for a balanced diet is, in any case, usually vastly overstated. Occasionally, someone's diet is grossly deficient in a particular vitamin, in which case it is possible to develop a deficiency disease. However, such diseases are almost unheard of in developed societies today. The one exception is rickets, which results from vitamin D deficiency. Even then, this is rarely due to poor diet but because children are not getting enough sunlight, which enables the skin to produce the vitamin. It is worth noting that the obsession with treating normal exposure to sunshine as a risk factor for skin cancer doesn't help, especially in such grey climates as the UK. For example, in some northern British cities, children have been provided with vitamin D supplements to deal with this in recent years.

In the badly-nourished developing world, on the other hand, deficiencies of iron (which causes anaemia) and vitamin A (which can cause blindness) are significant and serious problems. For all the hand-wringing about our so-called junk diets, the overwhelming majority of people in the developed world eat perfectly adequate diets from a health point of view. Indeed, according to figures from the Department of Environment, Food and Rural Affairs (Defra), published in *Family Food 2008*, UK consumers on average easily meet guideline intakes for most nutrients and come very close to the recommended amounts for the rest. Our diets may not always be optimal, from a nutritional point of view, but the vast majority of people eat food that is perfectly adequate to meet their body's needs.

Perhaps the problem is that our junk food diets are making us fat. However, *Family Food 2008* suggests that average energy intake is 2,276 calories per day, of which only about 10 per cent comes from meals eaten out. These calorie intakes suggest we are not exactly stuffing our faces. The usual guidelines for energy intake are 2,500 calories per day for men and 2,000 calories for women. On that basis, the current figures would appear to be pretty much exactly in line with that guidance. What precisely has caused the current rise in obesity rates is the subject of great debate (more of that in the next chapter); the usual pat explanations about eating too much or exercising too little don't really fit the evidence.

Ah, but maybe it's the 'additives' that are killing us. In Europe, there is a system of numbering commonly used food additives (there are hundreds of them). Yet as food writer and TV chef Stefan Gates shows in his book on the subject, most of the chemicals that are designated with 'E' numbers under this system are either naturally occurring in our food, and even in our bodies, or are absolutely essential to keeping our food free of dangerous infection.[5]

A particularly good example of a misplaced scare about an additive is monosodium glutamate (MSG). This is a much reviled flavour enhancer accused of causing all sorts of allergic reactions (with little evidence when properly tested). But as Gates explains, alongside our basic tastes of sweet, salt, sour and bitter, a fifth taste was discovered about 100 years ago: 'umami'. It is perhaps best summed up as 'savouriness' and is actually the taste of … glutamate. In fact, glutamate is central to making lots of food taste really good. Parmesan and other cheeses, tomatoes, mushrooms, soy sauce and lots of other very important foods contain loads of glutamate. In fact, our bodies naturally produce about 50 grams of it everyday.

There are, perhaps, a handful of food colours that could be phased out with little harm to our food or our health. Everything else on that long list of additives is well worth keeping.

[5]   Gates, S. (2010) *Stefan Gates on E Numbers*

In other words, the accusation that junk food is killing us seems wide of the mark. The diets of people in the developed world look pretty good in comparison to those in the developing world, to our diets in the not-too-distant past, and to health guidelines.

Good food, bad food

So if health worries cannot explain the notion of 'junk food', what can? How should we judge food? There's a lot of takeaway food that is, for various reasons, simply not very pleasant to eat. It may be made with very little care and attention from cheap ingredients. So, it is quite right and proper to make aesthetic judgements of this kind. If it doesn't taste good, don't buy it again.

That said, there is a difference between making a broad judgement about the merits of a particular food and an individual making a subjective judgement at any specific time: one man's meat is another man's poison, as the old saying goes. I spent most of the Nineties living in Edinburgh, where one of the most common sights in chip shops and supermarkets is the scotch pie, an unappealingly grey splodge of minced lamb and seasoning encased in crusty pastry. Having tried one, sober, I couldn't see why anybody would choose to eat one without a gun pointed at their head. Then, in the early hours of New Year's Day, having celebrated Hogmanay with a few drinks and much snogging of strangers on the city's Royal Mile, I joined the queue at a nearby chip shop only to find the last things available to eat were two scotch pies. In desperation, I bought them. But in my mildly inebriated state, with a severe case of the 'beer munchies', these two pies now seemed to be simply The Greatest Things I Had Ever Eaten. As another wise old saying puts it, 'hunger is the best sauce'.

There's a time and a place for almost any food. To use a musical analogy: Beethoven's Third Symphony is a landmark in musical history, marking the bridge between the earlier classical period and the romantic style that would dominate the nineteenth century. It is an ambitious piece that is much longer than previous symphonies and with an enormous emotional range. It is, objectively, a great piece of music. 'Agadoo', a novelty song by Black Lace, is an awful piece of music based on a cringeworthy dance routine. In 2003, *Q* magazine rated it the worst song ever: 'It sounded like the school disco you were forced to attend, your middle-aged relatives forming a conga at a wedding party, a travelling DJ act based in Wolverhampton, every party cliché you ever heard'.

But in the final throes of a drunken wedding reception, you wouldn't want the DJ to pop Beethoven on the turntable. You'd want the cringeworthy novelty song. And so it is with food. Even the most apparently trashy food has its place. It is perfectly possible to recognise that the food served by Gordon Ramsay, Heston Blumenthal or Michel Roux Jr—based on centuries of culinary history, years of personal training and experimentation, and the finest ingredients money can buy—is superior to fast food. The size of the bill would be indication enough. But it is still the case that sometimes a burger is absolutely the best thing to eat at that moment.

In any case, as Anthony Bourdain declares in his 2010 book, *Medium Raw*:

> I believe that the great American hamburger is a thing of beauty, its simple charms noble and pristine. The basic recipe — ground beef, salt and pepper, formed into a patty, grilled or seared on a griddle, then nestled between two halves of a bun, usually but not necessarily accompanied by lettuce, a tomato slice, and some ketchup—is to my mind, unimprovable by man or God.

Junk food for junk people?

I would argue that the division between junk food and real food has far more to do with a combination of middle-class angst and plain old-fashioned snobbery than anything else. To a degree, this is merely an expression of an age-old desire to mark out one's status by possessing that which others cannot afford.

Take bread. For centuries, it was the case that brown
bread was poor man's food. In her history of food fakery,
Swindled, Bee Wilson describes how a poor British wheat
harvest in 1756 drove Parliament to authorise a 'Standard'
bread, made with more bran than usual to make the most of
the nutrition available, and it was actually a little cheaper.
'To modern tastes, this bread sounds wholesome and good,
if a little worthy. But it wasn't popular then. People associated bran-rich bread with poverty. They wanted bread that
was whiter than white... Almost no one wanted to be the
sort of person who ate brown bread'. The result was the
excessive adulteration of bread with a white aluminium salt
called alum, producing an unpleasant tasting loaf and
sparking one of the earliest food panics.[6]

Jane Fearnley-Whittingstall's history of Britain's Second
World War Ministry of Food describes a similar situation,
when rationing meant that the only food available was the
wholemeal 'National Loaf'. It might have been seen as more
nutritious—wholemeal bread certainly seems to retain
more of the goodness of the wheat—but that doesn't mean
that people enjoyed it. Fearnley-Whittingstall notes that
'when white bread finally appeared again in the 1950s,
[people] were overjoyed'.[7]

Yet wholemeal bread is now highly prized, at least
among the middle classes. White bread still outsells brown
or wholemeal bread by a ratio of nearly two to one, according to *Family Food 2008*, but it is *panis non gratus* for the chat-
tering classes. In the *Guardian*, former public schoolboy
Oliver Thring describes the experience of eating 'bad bread'
for the first time in years: 'On the palate, cheap bread feels
like a kind of fungus, a pappy, vaguely elastic, glutinous,
gluey foam. It coats the roof of your mouth like an oral infection. It feels as though you could lag a loft with it. It's horri-
ble, as dry and refined as an art historian.'[8] You certainly

---

[6]   Wilson, B. (2008) *Swindled: From Poisonous Sweets to Counterfeit Coffee
        – The Dark History of the Food Cheats*
[7]   Fearnley-Whittingstall, J. (2010) *Ministry of Food: Thrifty Wartime
        Ways to Feed Your Family Today*
[8]   Consider cheap white bread, *Guardian*, 13 July 2010

need to be of a certain excitable disposition to get this hot under the collar about supermarket bread.

But the modern discussion of 'junk', processed and convenience food reveals a lot more than mere status seeking. Dismissing someone directly on the basis of social class is these days usually deemed unacceptable: it is done in a more coded fashion, including through the prism of diet. Right-thinking people eat in a certain way, generally some dreadful permutation of local, organic, minimally processed food. Wherever possible, they know the names of the baker, butcher and farmer. They, the Other, eat the cheap, processed, convenient products of industrialised food.

This dichotomy was clearly revealed in the reaction to a recent book by Delia Smith: *How to Cheat at Cooking*, an update of a book originally written in the early 1970s. Smith — truly the face of British TV cookery for decades whose books are like bibles to millions of (mostly) women — wanted to try to find a way to encourage people to cook more, even when they had relatively little time. Her method was to introduce into her recipes one or two time-saving, off-the-shelf convenience ingredients.

In the introduction to the book, Smith says that 'if you short-circuit some of the accepted rules of cooking and are willing to explore alternatives by adding the cheating element, you can discover a better and easier way of coping when there's not much available time'. She adds: 'Being a serious cheat can be very liberating. Without specific skills or precious time you can, whenever you want, produce spontaneous good food that's fun to prepare and free from anxiety.' That meant using things like frozen mashed potato or a ready-made sauce while still using fresh ingredients that needed little preparation.

Smith might have expected praise for this effort to get the nation cooking. Instead, the foodie commentariat had a hissy fit. Alex Renton, writing in the *Guardian*, explained how he and his wife had burned their copies of Smith's *How to Cook* after watching the TV series that accompanied *How to Cheat at Cooking*. Then, bringing together the full litany of crimes that processed food is apparently guilty of, Renton wailed:

> It's not just that the pre-prepared food Delia is flogging is an environmental nasty — in all its unnecessary processing, packaging and transport. Or that such stuff props up the 'value-adding' idiocies of the food-industry giants, which have brought them vast profit at the expense of farmers and traditional producers. It's more that just as the nation started to eat better, she's asking it to eat worse again. And that really is selling out.[9]

In a follow-up to this article a year later, Renton defended his position. Suggesting that Smith's decision to promote processed ingredients was as bad as Gandhi suggesting that punching people was okay after all, Renton wrote:

> Now, if you think that analogy is too much, you and I have a fundamental difference. You don't believe, as I do, that how we buy and use food is a moral issue. Or that processed and 'convenience' food sold at absurd prices by the big corporations that Delia now supports has done great damage to our society — to the rural economy, our health, and the environment — and that most of the harm has been done to the poorest people.[10]

(Not that the dangers of selling cheap ingredients at 'absurd' prices ever stopped anyone at a farmers' market flogging organic pork in a bun for four pounds a time.) I doubt that Delia Smith cared very much about the criticism: the book sold by the truckload. But her book was like an attack on the very identity of the chatterati. We are told that food must be healthy and wholesome, authentic and ethical. Simply feeding people tasty food with a minimum of fuss — to ignore the rules of these latter-day Pharisees — was simply beyond the pale. In the eyes of such foodies, it is these rules that separate Us from Them.

In the past, such middle-class haughtiness could have been quietly ignored. It would not have made any great impact on everyday life. But the collapse of traditional political and social solidarities, and the end of class politics, has left society more atomised and receptive to the fears and

[9]   Delia goes to the Dark Side, *Guardian*, 11 March 2008
[10]   My hounding by the Delia priesthood, *Guardian*, 17 March 2009

prejudices of the petit bourgeoisie. All the major political parties are middle-class now; and individualistic, fearful-of-the-future, chav-bashing, anti-consumption ideas are beamed to us 24/7 through the media with little contestation.

A.A. Gill, food critic for *The Sunday Times*, summed this up well in relation to the debate about organic food:

> What I really mind about all this is that organic is making food into a class issue. Organic brings back this prewar system of posh, politically correct food for Notting Hill people, and filthy, rubbish chemical food for filthy, rubbish chemical people. Either you are a nice organic person or you are a filthy, overweight McDonald's person. I find that really obscene. It has very little to do with food and a lot to do with weird snobbery.[11]

When we take the snobbery and prejudice out of our approach to food, it is much easier to see what is good and bad. Whether a particular food is 'natural', 'local' or 'organic' has precisely zero bearing on whether it is good. From a health point of view, by far the most important thing is to eat enough; a semblance of variety is probably beneficial, too. Otherwise, the only worthwhile question is whether or not something is pleasant to eat.

[11] Organic food has no health benefits, say officials, *The Sunday Times*, 2 August 2009

Chapter Four

Fat chance:
The obesity panic

We cannot afford not to act [on obesity]. For the first time we are clear about the magnitude of the problem. We are facing a potential crisis on the scale of climate change and it is in everybody's interest to turn things round. We will succeed only if the problem is recognised, owned and addressed at every level in every part of society.

Alan Johnson, health secretary for England, 2007

We are now in a situation where levels of childhood obesity will lead to the first cut in life expectancy for 200 years. These children are likely to die before their parents.

Colin Waine, chair of the UK National Obesity Forum, 2007

When a three-year-old girl who weighs 40 kilograms dies of heart failure brought on by obesity, you know her parents are guilty of gross child abuse...

Miranda Devine, Sydney Morning Herald, 2004

The surge of obesity among children, in short, presages a global explosion of illnesses that will drain economies, create enormous suffering and cause millions of premature deaths.

Madeleine Nash, Time, 2003

Perhaps the biggest issue relating to food in recent years has been obesity. As our waistlines have expanded, countless voices in the media, campaign groups, medical charities and government have warned us that we face disaster if we don't stop getting fatter.

Health secretary Alan Johnson's warning was made in advance of a report by the UK government's Foresight unit

entitled *Tackling Obesities: Future Choices*. The report itself
makes heavy reading. The summary of key findings notes:

> In recent years Britain has become a nation where over-
> weight is the norm. The rate of increase in overweight and
> obesity, in children and adults, is striking. By 2050, Fore-
> sight modelling indicates that 60 per cent of adult men, 50
> per cent of adult women and about 25 per cent of all chil-
> dren under 16 could be obese. Obesity increases the risk of
> a range of chronic diseases, particularly type-2 diabetes,
> stroke and coronary heart disease and also cancer and
> arthritis. The NHS costs attributable to overweight and
> obesity are projected to double to £10 billion per year by
> 2050. The wider costs to society and business are estimated
> to reach £49.9 billion per year (at today's prices).

The impact of rising obesity is even greater on the other
side of the Atlantic. In 2004, the US health secretary Tommy
Thompson presented figures from the Centers for Disease
Control and Prevention (CDC) suggesting that 400,000
Americans died each year due to their excess weight. Obesity is now frequently described as being right up there with
cigarette smoking as the world's biggest 'preventable'
cause of death.

Nor is this a problem confined to snack-scoffing couch
potatoes in the developed world. As a factsheet produced
by the World Health Organisation notes:

> Globally, there are more than one billion overweight
> adults, at least 300million of them obese; obesity and over-
> weight pose a major risk for chronic diseases, including
> type-2 diabetes, cardiovascular disease, hypertension and
> stroke, and certain forms of cancer; the key causes are
> increased consumption of energy-dense foods high in satu-
> rated fats and sugars, and reduced physical activity.[1]

Thou shalt be thin — or else

But if obesity is widely proclaimed to have devastating
health consequences, the reaction to obesity is pretty bad,
too. For example, in 2007, the mother of eight-year-old
Conor McCreadie from Newcastle in north-east England
was threatened with having her son removed from her

---

[1]   *Obesity and Overweight*, World Health Organisation, 2003

home because of his size. In 2009, seven children from a family in Dundee, Scotland, were removed from their home, with the children's weights being a major factor in the decision. The family's lawyer told the *Daily Mail* that the children's panel that decided upon the action had been 'very influenced by the social workers' recommendations ... The family is not being helped here, they have been systematically bullied and disempowered'.

In his 2004 book *The Obesity Myth*, the American commentator and lawyer Paul Campos describes the removal of a three-year-old child, Anamarie Regino, from her parents in New Mexico. The child ballooned to a weight of 130 pounds (59 kilogrammes), but doctors could not settle on any diagnosis of the problem, and nor could they find any reason why the child was in any immediate health danger. Yet the authorities assumed that she was being force-fed, possibly by a psychologically disturbed mother. (There was no evidence for that assumption, either). Eventually, little Anamarie did lose some weight thanks to a very extensive programme of diet and exercise. But Campos argues that the case says 'a great deal about the hysteria that fat elicits among so many doctors, social workers, and other members of helping professions'.

A feature in the *Albuquerque Journal* in March 2010 suggested that Anamarie is still struggling with her weight.[2] By then aged 12, standing five feet three inches tall and weighing over 300 pounds, Anamarie had a body mass index (BMI) of around 55. Doctors have still not been able to explain why she is so large.

Because obesity is deemed to be self-inflicted, obese people are in danger of being treated as second-class citizens when it comes to healthcare. In 2005, East Suffolk primary care trust in eastern England began to refuse hip and knee replacement operations to those classified as clinically obese. Brian Keeble, director of public health, said: 'We can-

---

[2]   Nine Years Ago, the State Took Custody of 3-Year-Old Ana Because of Her Weight; She Still Faces Challenges Today, *Alberquerque Journal*, 28 February 2010

not pretend that this [decision] wasn't stimulated by the pressing financial problems of the NHS in East Suffolk'.[3]

In 2011, NHS North Yorkshire and York announced it would stop patients who smoke, and those with a body mass index of more than 35, from having routine hip and knee surgeries because their unhealthy lifestyles allegedly lower the chance of the operations' 'success'. The motive for this rationing may have been 'unashamedly financial', but the fact that obesity could be used to justify such a refusal to operate in a system that is supposed to provide healthcare for all shows how far the obesity panic has gone.

Threats to obese people have reached the workplace, too. In Japan, a law came into force in 2008 requiring companies and local authorities to check the waist measurements of everyone aged 40 to 74 years. It follows concern about meta-bolic syndrome — a set of symptoms including high choles-terol, high blood pressure, obesity and diabetes — which the Japanese, with their habit of half-borrowing English words, have dubbed *metabo*. Those men whose waist exceeds 33.5 inches, or women whose waist exceeds 35.4 inches, will be given three months to get in shape, or face a further six months of health re-education. Companies that employ such people will be fined.[4]

If we cannot be trusted to do the right thing about our diets, governments are increasingly willing to listen to more direct interventions. Denmark has increased taxes on ice cream, chocolate, sweets and sugary soft drinks. There are soda taxes in 33 US states, although the tax rates are cur-rently pretty low. There has been talk, briefly, of a federal soda tax to help finance health-care reform.

New York mayor Michael Bloomberg has implemented a regulation that forces restaurants to display the calorie count of food items, something the current coalition gov-ernment in the UK has announced it will emulate. In the UK, there is also an ongoing debate about the merits of 'traffic

---

[3]   NHS cash crisis bars knee and hip replacements for obese, *Guardian*, 23 November 2005
[4]   Metabo tightens belts in land of rising tum, *Scotsman*, 15 June 2008

light' labelling for supermarket foods, with a 'red' label meaning that a food should be avoided.

These are merely some of the official reactions to obesity. Popular culture is full of examples of the obese being bashed or guilt-tripped about their weight. Take a documentary shown on UK digital TV channel More4 in 2006, entitled *Tax the Fat*. The presenter, restaurant critic Giles Coren, argued in an accompanying newspaper article:

> [T]he vast majority of chubbies in Britain are big because they lack the willpower or incentive to maintain a healthier lifestyle. We're paying for their self-indulgence. And I'm sorry, but I just don't think it's fair. Smokers are expected to pay vast amount in tax to fund their habit. Boozers are taxed in the same way; gamblers, too... The time has come to tax the fat.

Coren did not mean dietary fat—he meant fat people themselves. Perhaps the governor of Arizona, Jan Brewer, was watching. In April 2011, Brewer proposed a $50 top-up fee for Medicare receeipients who are obese, who smoke, or who are diabetic.[5]

Elsewhere on British TV, we've been treated to a 'feast' of obesity-related shows, from the poisonous moral blackmail of *You Are What You Eat* and *Honey We're Killing the Kids* (whose presenter, Kris Murrin, is now a UK government advisor), through the point-and-laugh so-called therapy of *Supersize vs Superskinny*, to watching overweight C-list personalities being humiliated in *Celebrity Fit Club* or ordinary people receiving the same treatment in *The Biggest Loser*.

How BMI couldn't Be More Imprecise

All this might make sense if the official advice on how to tackle obesity was based on a clear understanding of what makes us fat and provided clear, effective methods to tackle the problem. Sadly, it does not.

As the WHO factsheet cited above notes, the prevalence of 'overweight' and 'obesity' is measured by using a form of height-to-weight ratio called body mass index (BMI). BMI is

[5]   Reports: Arizona governor proposes obesity fee for Medicaid patients, *Orlando Sentinel*, 1 April 2011

a fairly crude way of assessing fatness first proposed by a Belgian mathematician, Adolphe Quetelet, in 1832. It is defined as a person's weight in kilogrammes divided by their height in metres squared (kg/m2). BMI only gained popularity after the well-known American medical researcher, Ancel Keys — who also popularised the idea that cholesterol causes heart disease — in 1972 proposed BMI as the best way of quickly assessing fatness.

In 1985, the US National Institutes for Health (NIH) established cut-off points for weight and health, based on BMI. Now BMI had the force of official backing. As a means of giving health authorities a rough idea of how our bodies are changing at the level of populations, BMI is crude but has the merit of simplicity. However, when applied to individuals, it has the potential to be downright distorting.

Currently, the following categories for BMI are widely recognised:

BMI range	Description	Weight at average UK height — male	Weight at average UK height — female
Less than 18.5	Underweight	Less than 57kg (125 pounds)	Less than 50kg (112 pounds)
18.5–25	Normal/ideal weight	Up to 77kg (168 pounds)	Up to 67kg (148 pounds)
25–30	Overweight	Up to 92kg (202 pounds)	Up to 81kg (178 pounds)
30–40	Obese	Up to 122 kg (270 pounds)	Up to 108kg (237 pounds)
More than 40	Morbidly obese		

However, there are problems with BMI as a way of measuring fatness and predicting health outcomes.

Firstly, BMI makes no distinction between fat and muscle mass. So someone who has been hitting the gym could qualify as overweight or obese despite having very little body fat. Handsome leading men like George Clooney, Brad Pitt and Matt Damon would qualify as overweight. Many sportsmen in peak condition would qualify as overweight or obese. For his famous 'Rumble in the Jungle' fight with George Foreman in 1974, Muhammad Ali – who would be regarded as relatively light by modern heavyweight standards – had a BMI of about 27, comfortably overweight using the standard definition. When a later heavyweight champ, Lennox Lewis – in the best shape of his life – fought Mike Tyson in 2002, he was borderline obese in terms of his BMI.

Conversely, people who apparently fall within the 'normal' or 'ideal' BMI category may be relatively unfit and carrying more body fat than someone who is regarded as overweight.

Secondly, BMI is blind to where fat is stored on the body, which some researchers and doctors – rightly or wrongly – believe may be crucial in determining whether that fat represents a health problem or not. Men, for example, seem to have a propensity to store fat around their waists while women store fat more evenly on their hips and breasts, too. Various attempts to account for this – by using waist measurement as a measure of obesity along with, or in place of, BMI – have been made, though the evidence is shaky that these are really any better as a measure of future health risk. A study published in *The Lancet* in 2011 suggests that waist size, hip-to-waist ratio and a variety of other measures are pretty poor at predicting who will suffer ill-health – suggesting that where fat is stored in the body may not be all that important.[6]

Thirdly, BMI gives a pseudo-scientific precision to the notion that carrying a bit of extra weight is going to kill you. In truth, the relationship between BMI and ill-health is more complicated. For example, after the US health secretary

---

[6]   *The Lancet*, Volume 377, Issue 9771, Pages 1085–1095, 26 March 2011

Tommy Thompson declared that 400,000 people died each year in the US from obesity, senior statisticians at CDC re-analysed the statistics and concluded that the figure was more like 25,000 deaths per year. This remarkable difference came about in large part because those in the 'overweight' category actually had longer life expectancies than those of 'normal' weight. Indeed, according to those revised figures, there is little difference in mortality between people in the 'normal', 'overweight' and 'mildly obese' categories. Only where individuals are either very underweight or very overweight is there a significant rise in mortality.

The US and UK authorities would have us believe that obesity itself should be regarded as a disease which, if not treated, will lead to other serious illnesses and a premature death. The simple formula, reflected in the WHO quote above, is that we're either eating too much or exercising too little and if we merely change these habits then we'll lose weight and everything will be hunky dory. The evidence, however, does not support such a simple conclusion.

There is no space here to discuss fully all the contradictory evidence about obesity. However, it is worth asking a few awkward questions about the way the relationship between our waistlines and our health is presented to us.

Bigger bellies, longer lives

It is certainly true that body weight has been on the rise for a while. Katherine Flegal, the senior researcher at the CDC who led the revision of Tommy Thompson's figures, has also noted elsewhere the sharp rise in the rate of people who were overweight or obese in the late 1980s. For example, in 1960, women aged 20 to 29 years old weighed, on average, 128 pounds (about 58 kg). By 2000, the average weight of that age group had risen to 157 pounds (just over 71kg). Over the same period, the weight of women in the 40 to 49 age group rose from 142 pounds (65kg) to 169 pounds (77kg). A similar leap has been seen in the UK: one in 10 adults was obese 30 years ago; today the figure is closer to one in four.

However, the weight gain may have been going on for even longer. In a paper in 2010, John Komlos and Marek Brabec use a range of sources to suggest that Americans, at least, have been getting fatter for 100 years and for many groups in society a lot of this weight gain occurred before the first official surveys were taken at the end of the 1950s.[7]

Rising life expectancy, however, has gone hand in hand with rising body weight. For example, as a comparison with Brabec and Komlos' observations, life expectancy in the US rose from 49.2 years at the start of the twentieth century to 68.1 years by the middle of the century and 77.5 years by 2003. That should at least suggest a little scepticism about the idea of an 'obesity timebomb' is in order.

Indeed, running alongside concerns about obesity causing us to die young is the ongoing worry that so many people will live to a ripe old age that the current arrangements for pensions will simply collapse. In December 2010, a report suggested that one in six individuals currently alive in the UK will live to be 100 years old. These two panics — the obesity timebomb and the pensions timebomb — seem to be contradictory.

Nonetheless, our waistlines have been expanding, and for very overweight people this seems to be associated with chronic health problems. What is causing this society-wide change in our body shapes?

Eat less, move more?

This is where things get really tricky. The official answer is based on the principle of the conservation of energy or, to put it another way, energy in must equal energy out. Therefore, the calories in our food, minus the calories we burn up with our metabolism and physical activity, equals the amount of fat we will store. To lose fat, therefore, we simply need to eat less or exercise more. Individual experience would seem to bear this out. If you are able, through force of

---

[7]   Komlos, J., Brabec, M. (2010) The Trend of Mean BMI Values of US Adults, Birth Cohorts 1882–1986 Indicates that the Obesity Epidemic Began Earlier than Hitherto Thought, *NBER Working Paper No. 15862*

will, to eat less over a long period of time, or exercise more without compensating for it by eating more, you seem to lose weight. So surely it is just a matter of personal discipline?

Yet even people who try *really* hard to lose weight usually find that their weight rebounds quickly after they stop whatever diet they were on — generally after months of ignoring hunger pangs. No matter what diet you examine — from Weight Watchers to the Cabbage Soup Diet and everything in between — the most striking finding is not that some diets are better than others but that pretty much all diets are abject failures at facilitating long-term, sustained weight loss. (Rather more worryingly, as *Diet Nation* authors Patrick Basham and John Luik have pointed out, this kind of yo-yo dieting appears to be associated with lower life expectancy than simply staying fat.[8] So much for healthy living.)

The argument put forward by the *Foresight* report is, at least, a little less moralistic than an obsession with our apparent personal weakness:

> Although personal responsibility plays a crucial part in weight gain, human biology is being overwhelmed by the effects of today's 'obesogenic' environment, with its abundance of energy-dense food, motorised transport and sedentary lifestyles. As a result, the people of the UK are inexorably becoming heavier simply by living in the Britain of today. This process has been coined 'passive obesity'. Some members of the population, including the most disadvantaged, are especially vulnerable to the conditions.[9]

The upshot is a call for ever more government intervention, going beyond simply the usual nannyish nagging.

Yet the debate about diet and exercise actually seems to be chasing its own tail. As the Australian academic Michael Gard told me in an interview in 2005:

> I had been doing some work on the side, looking into claims being made about obesity, such as that physical activity levels are declining. And I kept coming across

[8] Is dieting good for you? *spiked*, 22 March 2007
[9] Tackling Obesity: Future Choices, *Foresight*, 2007
http://bit.ly/i61ltu

statements like 'Of course, we have no conclusive proof …
but we know physical activity must be going down',
throughout the scientific literature.[10]

Yet in *The Obesity Epidemic*, Gard and his co-author Jan
Wright note that this kind of assumption is endemic in the
obesity literature. Studies show calorie intake to be falling
in recent decades, so it is assumed that physical activity
must be falling even faster to explain the rise of obesity. But
studies of physical activity find no change over time (and
for some groups, like middle-class women, greater access to
sport suggests it may well have increased), leaving
researchers to assume that our expanding waistlines are a
product of increasingly gluttonous tendencies.

In fact, it is striking just how bad the simple expenditure
of calories is at helping us to lose weight. A common com-
plaint among marathon runners, for example, is that after
hundreds of miles of training and a feat of endurance —
running 26 miles non-stop — they very often lose little or no
weight. Yet our apparently sedentary lifestyles are constantly held up as a reason for the rise of obesity.[11]

In short, Gard and Wright conclude that these studies
have taught us nothing useful about why obesity rates have
risen or what we might do about it. So fixated are researchers with the idea that obesity must be caused by an imbalance between calories ingested and calories expended that
they cannot see that this way of looking at the problem has
failed to explain anything. It is rather like trying to explain
why someone is an alcoholic by concluding that they drink
too much. That's not an explanation, it is merely restating
the problem.

It may be that the mainstream presentation of obesity gets
the cart before the horse. The calories in / calories out view
must be correct to satisfy a basic law of physics: the conservation of energy. But as the American science writer Gary
Taubes points out, cause and effect could be the other way
round: we start eating more or moving around less because

[10]   Fat and Fiction, *spiked*, 10 June 2005
[11]   For a fuller discussion of this point, see Weight loss: the futility of the
       exercise, *spiked*, 12 April 2011

of some internal, metabolic change. Taubes makes the comparison with children growing: during the adolescent growth-spurt, children will often start eating far more food than before. Do they then get taller because they suddenly eat more? Hardly. Rather, they eat more because their bodies are growing and demanding more food. Could this not also apply to the laying down of fat?

Taubes argues that it is our high-carbohydrate diets—much encouraged by the relentless health advice to eat low-fat diets—that have perversely caused us to pile on the pounds in recent years. It's an interesting theory, and in his book *Good Calories, Bad Calories*, Taubes provides an impressive array of detail on why the changing balance of our diets could be the problem. You don't need to be a junk-food junkie either: if you cut out fat, but you still consume enough calories to maintain health, that shortfall must be made up mostly or totally by eating more carbs.

Taubes notes that the one hormone that regulates whether our bodies store fat or not is insulin. And what causes insulin levels to rise? The consumption of carbohydrates. The principle can be seen in reverse with type-1 diabetics: those whose bodies produce little or no insulin and must inject insulin to control their blood sugar. In 2007, BBC News reported on a dangerous fashion among young diabetics to skip their insulin injections in order to lose weight. No insulin means no fat can be stored, resulting in weight loss. The downside is a very serious risk of blindness and various other problems.[12]

If obesity was simply a matter of too much energy in, or not enough energy out, then everyone would put on weight to the same degree no matter what they consumed. However, this isn't the case.

In his film, *Super Size Me*, American comedian Morgan Spurlock tried eating nothing but McDonald's food for a month and, whenever it was offered to him, he ate the 'super size' option, often grossing out on 5,000 calories per day—roughly double the suggested intake for an adult

[12]   Diabetes eating disorder warning, BBC News, 4 July 2007

man. The result was that he piled on the pounds, felt dreadful, and his doctors told him that for a variety of measures like liver function he was making himself seriously ill.

Fredrik Nyström from the University of Linköping tried repeating Spurlock's idea with a group of university students, though not eating exclusively at McDonald's. The first thing that they found was that eating 5,000 calories a day is not easy — it takes hard work to force that much food down. Secondly, while everyone seemed to gain weight, for some people the weight gain was comparatively small — about five per cent — then plateaued. Only a small proportion of people gained a lot of weight, suggesting that some people have a propensity to gain weight but most achieve a steady state even with such enormous food intakes.[13]

In the 1960s, the University of Vermont researcher Ethan Sims gave convicts at Vermont State Prison first 4,000 calories a day and then later 5,000, 7,000 and even 10,000 calories per day (four times the recommended calorie intake, an enormous amount of food). Gary Taubes summarises Sims' results:

> Of his eight subjects that went 200 days on this mildly heroic regimen, two gained weight easily and six did not. One convict managed to gain less than 10 pounds after 30 weeks of forced gluttony (going from 134 pounds to 143). When the experiment ended, all the subjects 'lost weight readily'...[14]

These and other studies suggest that some members of society have a particular predisposition to pile on the pounds, perhaps as the result of a hormonal over-reaction to consuming carbohydrate, while the rest of the population will become mildly chubby at best. In turn, that suggests that the obesity panic is wrong-headed.

Instead of demanding that we all constantly monitor how much we eat, the health authorities would do better to take a serious look at the research evidence and try to find out why

[13]　For more on this study, see 'Only another 5500 calories to go...', *Guardian*, 7 September 2006

[14]　Quoted in Taubes, G. (2007) *Good Calories, Bad Calories*

some people get very fat. For a small proportion of people-
—perhaps two or three per cent in the UK—weight gain
becomes a significant problem, even if only in the sense that
carrying that much bulk around is so difficult. For the rest of
us, the moralising and lecturing provides no benefit at all
—just a bellyful of guilt and anxiety.

Chapter Five

Schooled in food panics

The school meals service in the UK had been in decline for decades before 2005. Then *Jamie's School Dinners*, a television series on Channel 4, turned school meals into a cause célèbre, which even featured as a major issue in that year's UK General Election. The events around the school dinners crusade illuminate many facets of society's eating disorder.

The idea of schools providing children with something good to eat every lunchtime — and perhaps at breakfast, too — seems like a fine idea. I was a double beneficiary of the school meals service: not only was my mum a school dinner lady, but I received free school meals, too. For a relatively hard-up family, a hot meal at school means one fewer meal to be paid for, while the breakfast club means mum and dad can get to work on time knowing that the kids are being taken care of. Nor is this simply a British phenomenon: one US author subtitled her book on school meals 'America's favourite welfare program'.

Providing meals in a school canteen is also a civilising thing to do. It is important for children to learn how to conduct themselves at the table, and school meals also offer an opportunity for adults and peers to encourage children to try new foods.

However, I would rather children ate takeaways or such unappetising offerings as 'turkey twizzlers' (the coils of minced turkey, fat and seasoning that achieved national notoriety in Britain's school dinners panic) than for society to keep up the moralistic scaremongering and instrumentalism that currently drives school-meals policy. Rather than presenting better school meals as an end in themselves, we've loaded all sorts of preoccupations on to them. And turning the provision of school meals from a catering issue into a crusade has had some pretty troubling side-effects.

We run the risk of placing too great a burden on school meals. We seem to believe that providing schoolchildren with a good meal can somehow solve all manner of wider problems. In reality, this fantasy has had markedly negative consequences for the school meals service, parental autonomy and the relationship between parents and schools.

School meals past

The school meals panic brought with it a nostalgic myth that there was some kind of 'Golden Age' of school dinners. There may have been more variety in the days when I was eating school meals and my mum was cooking them, but they were still mostly composed of stodge. We fondly remember the puddings: apple crumble, or the chocolate rice krispie things that disintegrated into your custard. But for every nostalgia-inducing entrée or dessert there was another which amounted to culinary torture: my primary school's foul-tasting braised liver put me off the idea of trying paté for years, and if many economy burgers today are of dubious origin, god only knows what went into a 'steaklet'.

School meals were created as an attempt to deal with the genuinely bad state of nutrition for many children. Back then, it was not so much a case of not eating quite the right balance of foods; some children were not getting enough to eat at all. In 1879, Manchester started to provide free school meals to badly-nourished children and there were various other attempts around the UK to provide meals for needy children over the subsequent 20 years.

However, the evidence was building that many working-class people simply did not have enough to eat, well illustrated by the surveys by Charles Booth and Seebohm

Rowntree in the late nineteenth and early twentieth century. The problem was further highlighted by the poor physical state of the potential recruits for the Boer War, which meant that in some geographical areas two thirds of applicants were deemed unfit to fight. Negative publicity about these things, alongside pressure from 29 MPs elected in 1906 representing the recently formed Labour Party, led the Liberal government to allow local authorities to provide food to schoolchildren — though the provision of such meals was not, at this time, compulsory.

The 1921 Education Act set out the circumstances in which children should be provided with free school meals, but these were quickly rationed due to the rising cost, with the result that many children who should have received them did not. In 1936, for example, a survey of local education authorities found that only 2.7 per cent of children received free meals.

The circumstances of war, when women were required to do the work left by men who had gone off to fight, meant that children needed to be fed at midday by schools because they could not go home. As Penelope Hall notes: 'The "feeding centre" was gradually transformed into the "school canteen", and by February 1944 32.8 per cent of the number of pupils present were having dinners.'

If there was ever a 'Golden Age' of school meals, it began with the 1944 Education Act, which made it compulsory for local authorities to provide school meals, free of charge, to poorer children and at no more than the cost of raw ingredients to the rest. Free school milk was also provided from 1946 to all schoolchildren. In 1945, the minister of food, Lord Woolton, told the Warwickshire Women's Institute:

> The young need protection and it is proper that the state should take deliberate steps to give them opportunity... Feeding is not enough, it must be good feeding... This is a task that calls for the highest degree of scientific catering; it mustn't be left to chance.[1]

---

[1]   Quoted in Gillard, D. (2003) Food for thought: child nutrition, the school dinner and the food industry, *Forum*, Vol 45 No 3

That does not mean that all was well. By 1951, 49 per cent of pupils ate school meals and 84 per cent drank school milk. But they often did so in less than ideal circumstances, a situation summed up by Penelope Hall, prefiguring some modern concerns about ignorant parents and rushed meals:

> The primary aim of the school meals service is the adequate nutrition of all the nation's children, but it is intended to do more than this. The school meal is regarded in many quarters as an opportunity for social training, and for the inculcation of good food habits, both very important items in the education of all children, particularly perhaps in that of over-indulged only children, or those from homes where the mother's ignorance of food values is matched by her indifference to them.

Hall continues:

> If anything worthwhile is to be done in the way of social training however, the meals must be properly supervised, served in an orderly manner, preferably with the help of the children themselves, and eaten without haste in a happy atmosphere and pleasant surroundings. Unfortunately these conditions are not being fulfilled in many canteens to-day. Too often the premises are make-shift and overcrowded, the supervisors harassed, the meal bolted and the children hurried out to make room for a second batch. Shortages of premises, staff and equipment are largely responsible for this state of affairs, but until they are overcome the school meal cannot be fully effective as an integral part of the child's education.[2]

The unraveling of school food provision is often thought to have begun in 1970 when, as education secretary, Margaret Thatcher withdrew free school milk from school pupils aged seven to 11 (hence the chant, 'Thatcher, Thatcher, milk snatcher') and raised the cost of school meals. However, as Charles Webster points out, the process had actually started two years earlier under Harold Wilson's Labour government, when the cost of a meal went up from one shilling to one shilling and six pence — a 50 per cent rise. A further rise

---

[2]   Hall, M.P. (1963) *The Social Services of Modern England*

of three pence was implemented in 1969. Free school milk was removed from secondary schools in 1968.[3]

In 1980, Margaret Thatcher — then prime minister — started to run down the school meals service. Nutritional standards were scrapped and local authorities were only obliged to provide meals to poorer children. Competitive tendering meant that many school meals were 'contracted out' from local authorities to private contractors and the number of children eligible for free meals was further reduced by the Social Security Act 1986.

The school meals crusade

By the time Tony Blair's Labour government was elected in 1997, there was growing concern at the state of school meals and children's diets more generally. The Labour government did start to impose some basic guidelines limiting the number of times per week foods like chips and beans could be served in primary schools, and ensuring that fresh fruit was available at least twice per week. But these were food-based rather than nutrition-based standards.

While there had been campaigners around school meals before, like the Nottingham school cook Jeanette Orrey and the Child Poverty Action Group, the issue only really caught the imagination of the public — and, almost inevitably, the interest of politicians — after Jamie Oliver's television series in 2005.

Oliver went into a south London secondary school, Kidbrooke, with the aim of improving the quality of the lunches on offer. Oliver revealed that school meals no longer meant cooking from scratch with basic ingredients. Rather, packets of frozen meal elements like burgers and pizzas were simply opened, dumped into metal trays, and heated up. Oliver's aim was to revive the practice of cooking from fresh, on site. However, it quickly became apparent that producing a satisfying meal with ingredients that cost a

---

[3]   Webster, C. (1997) Government policy on school meals and welfare
      foods 1939-1970, in Smith, D.F. *Nutrition in Britain*

mere 37 pence per head was a challenge even for a superstar chef like Oliver.

Oliver also proved to be clueless about how to cater for hundreds of diners in a very short period of time. His food was too slow and too expensive. Worse, the pupils simply didn't fancy it — at least at first — which meant that much of it went to waste. Fortunately for Oliver, the school's catering manager (ie, head dinner lady) — the delightful, combative and mischievous Nora Sands — went out of her way to make the pilot scheme a success.

As the TV show presents it, take-up of the new-style meals started to increase thanks to a range of initiatives. Firstly, Oliver changed his menus to make some of the new food seem more familiar. Secondly, as schools were switched to the new menus, lessons and activities were created that helped to explain why the food was changing and to give children a sense of ownership of the process.

Nonetheless, persuading children to change their eating habits was ultimately down to time and the hard business of persuasion. When one boy at Kidbrooke, initially a new food refusenik, was asked by Oliver why he had started eating the meals, his answer was simple: 'Nora'. Having an adult persuade children to try something new — and keep nagging till they did — proved crucial.

However, there was one prophetic comment early in the series. When talking to one of the major catering companies, Scolarest, Oliver had insisted that the old 'junk' foods must be taken off the menu. The Scolarest rep warned that 'if you ban them completely and they don't recognise any foods on that menu, they just won't come in, they'll vote by their feet, and a lot of the vulnerable children will not have their free meal entitlement'.

Lo and behold, a major effect of Oliver's campaign was to drive parents and children away from school meals. Having been told that school food was killing their kids — an utterly overcooked claim — parents decided it would be wiser simply to give children packed lunches or money to buy takeaway food instead. A year after the series, officials in Gloucestershire, one of the first counties to make the switch to healthier dinners, had seen the numbers of primary-school children taking meals falling from 11,600 to 9,800 out of a total of 40,000 pupils. There was an even bigger decrease in Suffolk, where the total number of school meals served in the year after Jamie's School Dinners fell from 19,000 to 13,000.

In the country as a whole, 400,000 children had reportedly turned their backs on school meals — a 12.5 per cent fall — a decline which called into question the financial viability of some school meals services.

Blaming parents

Oliver's reaction was to slam parents who replaced the school dinner with a lunchbox. Packed lunches 'are the biggest evil. Even the best packed lunch is a shit packed lunch', he declared diplomatically.[4] The result was to turn teachers into 'lunchbox police' with nutritional guidelines set, not just for school meals, but for the food that parents decided was appropriate to put in lunchboxes, too. If that wasn't enough, some schools implemented 'lock-down' policies to prevent pupils from finding alternative sustenance in the local takeaways.

In Rotherham, the reorganisation of lunches at one school led to children struggling to get lunch before being sent back to the classroom — and they weren't too keen on the food being dished up anyway. Two mothers of pupils at the school, Julie Critchlow and Sam Walker, started to bring takeaway food to the school to push through the fence to the children. They soon became the targets of national vitriol.

Critchlow told *The Sun*:

> I started doing this for my kids and a couple of their friends, but every day more and more are wanting us to do the food run. We go up at 11 o'clock and take down orders through the fence. Then we go back at 1pm to deliver the food and give them their change. We're now delivering 50 to 60 meals a day and there are four of us doing it. We've no intention of stopping. We don't make a penny on it, we just

---

[4]   Jamie is back on the offensive over school dinners, *Independent on Sunday*, 2 April 2006

want the kids properly fed. They don't enjoy the school
food and the end result is they're starving.[5]

Walker told the paper: 'This is all down to Jamie Oliver. I
just don't like him and what he stands for. He's forcing our
kids to become more picky about their food'. Oliver's
spokesperson responded:

> If these mums want to effectively shorten the lives of their
> kids and others' kids, then that's down to them. What peo-
> ple don't realise is that junk food doesn't just help make our
> children fat, it's also a growing cause of malnourishment.
> Many kids just aren't getting the nutrition they need to
> grow healthily.

The Sun itself ran a cartoon in the same day's paper, presenting Walker and Critchlow in similar vein to *Viz* comic's Fat
Slags. As Brendan O'Neill noted at the time:

> Here, we can glimpse the reality and the fantasy of today's
> obesity panic. The reality is that people who eat 'junk food'
> are quite healthy and happy; the fantasy, as indulged by
> celeb chef Jamie Oliver, his supporters in government and
> both the broadsheet and tabloid media, is that people who
> eat junk food are immoral fat 'tossers' (in Oliver's words)
> who are beyond the bounds of civilised society.[6]

The school meals campaign has since started to leave its
mark beyond the school gate. In October 2010, a court ruled
that councils can take into account the health of schoolchildren when considering planning permission to takeaway
food shops. In future, it seems, permission may not be
granted for takeaways that are too close to schools. It seems
the government will have its way and children will eat the
'right thing' whether they like it or not.

Nor was it simply parents and pupils getting uppity.
School dinner ladies revolted against the longer hours they
were expected to work—often unpaid—to get the more
labour-intensive meals prepared. In May 2006, more than a
year after *Jamie's School Dinners*, there were rumblings of
strike action in London's school kitchens. Cathy Stewart, a

[5]   Sinner ladies sell kids junk food, *The Sun*, 16 September 2006
[6]   'Sinner Ladies': the fantasy and reality, *spiked,*18 September 2006

dinner lady in east London and a union representative told
the *New Statesman*:

> Overnight, we were expected to start seasoning meat and
> peeling hundreds of carrots — but that takes time and we're
> not being paid for it … They want dinner ladies to become
> professional chefs. But they won't give us the resources we
> need. We have outdated equipment and we don't have
> enough staff.[7]

The rotten ideas behind the school food debate

Jamie Oliver was hardly solely to blame for these negative
reactions. Though he did himself no favours with his capacity for the less-than-diplomatic quote, he was only representing a whole bunch of unhelpful attitudes that are
widely accepted in the modern debate about food.

One is the reaction against big business — even when
using large companies might be the best way to get things
done. For example, in the follow-up to the TV series, *Jamie's
Return to School Dinners*, Oliver tackled the problem of feeding children at a primary school in Lincolnshire — ironically,
the area of the country where Margaret Thatcher was born.
The school had no kitchen because of the cuts in school
meals in the past, so the children all ate packed lunches. Oliver decided that the only way around this problem was to
cook food at a local pub then ferry it to the school. Never
mind that the pub was so cramped that the chef was putting
pots of food on the floor to stir them. Moreover, the hygiene
standards required to provide pub grub and those
demanded when feeding hundreds of children are poles
apart.

The upshot was that a pub, which in no way was set up to
the high standards of school catering, was trying to prepare
food in less-than-ideal circumstances and losing money in
the process while parents were volunteering to ferry the
food from the pub to the school. That might have worked
with a bit of celebrity cajoling and a camera crew on hand,
but it was a situation unlikely to be sustained in the long
term. What was truly blinkered was Oliver's unwillingness

---

[7]   Jamie leaves a nasty aftertaste, *New Statesman*, 8 May 2006

to consider working with the kind of firms that do this type of catering on a grand scale. With a bit of imagination (and the expanded budget for ingredients that Oliver had wrung out of the government), a catering firm could have provided better meals. Instead, the small-is-beautiful, fresh-is-best prejudices of modern foodies meant that Oliver probably never even considered the possibility.

Another prejudice is the assumption that if children eat a diet of reheated food at school then they will never develop a taste for other foods. But childish conservatism when it comes to food does not mean that children won't learn to love a broader range of foods as adults. In an interview for *The Times* in 2009, Hugh Fearnley-Whittingstall—another campaigning chef, who came to fame for his eat-anything attitude, such as cooking up roadkill—described his own fussy childhood habits:

> The food I loved, I loved with passion. Findus Crispy Pancakes, boy did I love them. Fish fingers: completely addicted. Also my mum's spaghetti Bolognese. I used to be really fussy. There was a whole list of foods I wouldn't touch which definitely included mushrooms or tomatoes in any shape or form, except ketchup. Couldn't put them in my mouth without gagging.[8]

Never mind the 'junk' food: Oliver's school meals campaign was packed with junk ideas in desperate need of a pinch of salt—in both a literal and a metaphorical sense. Salt is now regarded in schools as something to be feared, like an unexploded bomb rather than an essential component of flavour. Even before Oliver's campaign, school catering assistants were told not to add salt to food. That made some sense when the processed products they were dishing up already included salt. But that wasn't the case with Oliver's offerings, and the salt rules became a source of considerable irritation to him when it came to trying to create alternative menus. The 2009 school meal guidelines also required the removal of salt from canteen tables. The fixation with salt is

[8]   Hugh Fearnley-Whittingstall makes it simple at River Cottage, *The Times* (London), 7 October 2009

strange, not least because the UK government's Scientific Advisory Committee on Nutrition reported in 2003:

> The evidence of a contribution from salt intake to raised blood pressure in children is limited and it is not clear whether sodium intake in isolation is a factor in the development of hypertension in the young which then tracks into adulthood. More work is needed in this area before firm conclusions can be drawn.[9]

The blanket ban on salt indicates how little the school meals crusade was motivated by genuine food standards: providing kids with a tasty meal.

We should also take a metaphorical pinch of salt in relation to the food panics and claims made about children's diets. One of the main drivers of the resurgent interest in school meals has been the talk of the 'obesity timebomb' discussed in chapter 4. In the TV show, Oliver suggested that this was the first generation expected to die before their parents (a claim he reworded for a later series, *Jamie's American Food Revolution*, as 'die at a younger age than their parents').

In reality, the current generation of children is almost certainly going to live significantly longer, on average, than their parents, regardless of the problem of obesity, because of a range of other factors from falling smoking rates to improvements in medicine.[10]

Moreover, to the extent that obesity is a problem, will providing one government-approved meal a day really solve it? Consider the assumption that if kids don't eat healthily when they are young, then they will simply carry on expanding throughout adulthood. In fact, the relationship between childhood obesity and long-term adult obesity is much weaker than that. Human bodies go through a lot of changes in the journey from childhood to adulthood, with the result that a lot of skinny kids (including me) get fatter in later life, while chubby children often become comparatively lean adults.

---

[9] *Salt and Health*, Scientific Advisory Committee on Nutrition, 2003
[10] For more discussion of life-expectancy trends, see Leon, D. (2011) Trends in European life expectancy: a salutary view, *International Journal of Epidemiology*

The population in the UK has been getting fatter gradually for decades, even during what many would see as the golden age of school meals. Yet this gradual fattening has coincided with an equally steady rise in life expectancies. That suggests that obesity is not a disease, and nor is it a death sentence. It also suggests that creating better school meals will do little to change matters.

Obesity was not the only 'porkie' that Oliver's series dished up. Another idea doing the rounds is that feeding children well at lunchtime will magically improve their performance in the classroom. Oliver's 'Feed Me Better' campaign manifesto stated:

> A lunchtime school dinner should give kids a third of their daily nutrition requirements. That's why it should be packed with not only fresh produce, but all the proteins, minerals and vitamins needed for health and growth. Diet also affects kids' behaviour, their physical and mental development, and their ability to learn — another good reason to ban the junk and go fresh and tasty.

The idea that kids are more 'manic' on a 'sugar rush' is popularly aired amongst parents and teachers alike. But it is reductionist to put the problems of schooling down to eating habits. Children are more than just the sum of their chemical inputs.

In some schools, changing the way that meals are provided seems to have had a broader positive impact. But it seems most likely that this came about because the emphasis on improving the food gave the schools a sense of collective purpose that may have been lacking previously. It seems rather insulting to reduce the efforts of teachers, parents and the local community to a question of how much vitamin C, iron or saturated fat a child is ingesting. Even the simple matter of sitting down to a proper meal with crockery and cutlery instead of being handed cheap food on a plastic tray in a manner more akin to a prison than a place of education must surely have some impact on pupils' perceptions of being at school.

Jamie's School Dinners also suggested that a better diet would reduce asthma attacks. I contacted Asthma UK, the leading charity for the condition in Britain, and was told that while the organisation recommends that asthma sufferers have a balanced diet, and that specific foods such as oily fish may be of some help, food is only occasionally mentioned as a trigger for attacks. The 'trigger' foods were as likely to be 'healthy', such as bananas or cheese, as they were to be processed. Asthma may occur in people with an allergy to a particular foodstuff, but as an article in the journal *Paediatrics* noted in 2003, 'chronic or isolated asthma or rhinitis induced by food is unusual'.

Perhaps the most lurid claim of the TV series was that grossly overweight children could end up vomiting their faeces. Is that really possible? Professor Roy Pounder of Royal Free and University College medical school told me at the time that it is possible to regurgitate barely digested food in severe cases of constipation — but it's extremely rare. This regurgitated food might look like faeces, but it's not. 'I'm just finishing 25 years at the Royal Free Hospital', he told me, 'and with simple constipation I don't think I've ever seen it. ... It's vanishingly unlikely for children to vomit from constipation. To reach the point of blocking to vomit, I would be looking for another reason for their vomiting'.

A better way forward for children's food

After *Jamie's School Dinners*, fewer children now eat school meals than before, contributing to the existing secular decline; parents and pupils are more tightly regulated about even the intimate business of deciding what to eat; and even local businesses can be shut down or refused licences to trade in the name of healthy eating. For all this, Oliver is lauded as 'Saint Jamie'. His motivation may have been a genuine desire to feed children better, but combined with the authoritarian streak of food campaigners and health watchdogs, the school meals campaign has only reduced personal freedom while having minimal benefit to the long-term health of children.

So what would I suggest? First of all, we need to be a lot more critical of certain health claims. The more shocking the claim, the more it needs to be carefully examined. Not only do such claims tend to be overblown, but the upshot of every health scare seems to be that someone needs to intervene more aggressively in the minutiae of our lives.

Secondly, feeding children must be seen first and foremost as a parental responsibility. The school meals service is a valuable thing, but it should be there to help parents, not become another stick with which to beat them. After all, it is parents who have to deal with their children's fussy eating habits while balancing family budgets. Teachers should be working hard to make sure that children can read, write and add up, not lecturing children and parents about chocolate bars and packets of Monster Munch.

Education budgets are under constant pressure. The first priority must be to improve the quality of learning, not eating. But if we decide to devote more resources to school meals, let's give children good meals because that's the right thing to do. We don't need to justify it by damning parents or pretending that eating certain kinds of food will save education and turn out model citizens.

Chapter Six

A smorgasbord of panics

Every day seems to bring a new panic about one food or another. Here's a quick, random sample: bacon and bladder cancer; beef and breast cancer; canned fish and premature birth; trans fats and heart disease; breakfast cereals and high blood pressure; food additives and hyperactivity; bottled water and cancer; processed food and mental illness...

The sheer volume of panics about what we eat and drink has got to the point where we barely notice them anymore. But they do have an insidious effect on how we treat food.

Pregnant women are both frequently the objects of this kind of scare and particularly susceptible to such scaremongering. Everything, it seems, that goes into a pregnant woman's mouth is bad for baby. One article on the BBC website warned pregnant women about 'weight gained during one pregnancy affecting the next one; drinking alcohol; blue cheese; soft cheese; shellfish; caffeine; bagged salad; coleslaw; cigarettes; flax seed; paté; liver; raw eggs; hot baths; lack of folic acid; too much exercise'.

A symptom of our societal eating disorder is the extent to which food is often presented, less as a source of sustenance and nutrition, but as a dangerous toxin. How did we get to this point? A quick look back over the past couple of decades reveals two particularly significant food panics, which greased the pan for our susceptibility to worries about anything we might want to eat.

Mad cows and Englishmen: the BSE panic

In 1986, the UK's Central Veterinary Laboratory formally identified a new cattle disease with distressing symptoms: disorientated, weak-limbed animals stumbling around for a few weeks before collapsing entirely. The disease was bovine spongiform encephalopathy (BSE), which in the UK directly killed 179,000 cattle and led to the culling of 4.4million, with the total cost of various interventions and compensation running to £5 billion.

The way in which the BSE crisis unfolded subsequently had a significant impact on food policy, going well beyond concerns over the safety of meat.

BSE was not the first disease of its kind. A similar disease — scrapie — has been known in sheep since the eighteenth century. Indeed, BSE was initially assumed to be scrapie that had managed to leap the species barrier from sheep to cattle. With hindsight, it seems that a few cases of BSE probably occurred in the 1970s, but were not identified as such. At first, nothing very much happened to respond to the outbreak, partly because the State Veterinary Service placed an embargo on public discussion of this new disease. However, by the end of 1987, the authorities suspected that the disease was being spread through food created from meat and bone from dead cattle that was treated, then recycled, as animal feed. This led to the popular idea that BSE was blowback for cost-cutting in the processing of cattle feed, fuelling concerns that short-term profit was trumping consumer safety.

It was assumed at the time that the disease had only just emerged, that it had come from sheep, and that changes to the way in which meat had been treated to create animal feed were responsible for allowing the infection to be transmitted. As it would later emerge, the disease was not entirely new and it did not come from sheep. Moreover, it transpired that the rendering process used in making cattle feed had never been capable of completely removing the infectious agent thought to be responsible — a kind of misshapen protein called a prion.

In 1988, a working party — the Southwood Committee — was set up to investigate the risks to human health of BSE. The report concluded that the risk of transmission of BSE to humans appeared remote and that 'it was most unlikely that BSE would have any implications for human health'. This assessment was based on the idea that BSE had derived from scrapie. Since humans hadn't been infected with scrapie in the previous 200 years, it was deemed unlikely that BSE would infect them, either.

As the animal epidemic progressed, new rules and regulations were introduced. Later in 1988, feed based on animal protein was banned and the decision was taken to slaughter all BSE-infected cattle. In 1989, beef offal was banned from baby food, restrictions on exports to Europe were introduced, and the use of cow brain and spinal cord was banned for human consumption. But the defining image of the whole 'mad cow' episode came in May 1990, when the agriculture secretary, John Selwyn Gummer, offered his daughter Cordelia a bite from a hamburger for the benefit of the gathered media. The message was that if the minister was confident enough to feed beef to his daughter, ordinary consumers should feel confident about eating it, too.

The turning point in the BSE crisis came when cases of what appeared to be a novel form of spongiform encephalopathy appeared in humans in 1995. Creutzfeldt-Jakob disease (CJD) is named after the two German neurologists who identified it and has been known since 1920. Its symptoms include dementia, memory loss and hallucinations along with loss of balance, rigid posture and seizures. CJD causes a few dozen cases in mostly older people each year. These new cases, while having many similarities to the 'sporadic' form of CJD, were distinct primarily because they were in much younger people, and these were classified as 'new variant CJD' (later, simply 'variant CJD' or vCJD).

In March 1996, the health secretary Stephen Dorrell announced in parliament that, in the absence of any alternative explanation, these cases were mostly likely to have been the result of exposure to BSE-infected beef products. Having been perhaps a little too willing to accept that BSE would be just like scrapie—a reasonable assumption, but not one based on any thorough scientific research—the authorities lurched violently the other way in making an announcement that created panic without achieving anything in terms of improving public safety.

As Dr Michael Fitzpatrick notes, Dorrell's announcement 'had no public health value: measures to prevent transmission of BSE to humans had already been introduced in 1988–89'.[1] What followed was a collapse in beef sales and an import ban by the European Union. Now obsessed with shutting down on even theoretical risks, sales of beef on the bone were banned in December 1997 and the ban remained in place for two years. Yet there remained considerable mystery as to how the disease might be transmitted and some doubt as to whether BSE really could be the causative factor, given the small number of cases and the fact that even long-standing vegetarians had succumbed.[2]

The advice that BSE was not a significant risk to humans had been given in good faith, and the numbers identified as suffering from vCJD were small. But that didn't prevented apocalyptic speculation about the long-term impact of vCJD based on models that produced wildly different estimates of deaths. A paper in 1997 in *Nature* offered a range of possible numbers of future cases from as little as 75 (if the disease's incubation period proved to be no more than 10 years) to 80,000 if the incubation period were 25 years;[3] others speculated about millions of deaths. Such widely differing and speculative figures were little use in planning, but did provide material for more 'shock horror' headlines.

The truth is, however, that the threatened vCJD epidemic has never happened. At the time of writing, a total of 171 deaths had been reported to the CJD surveillance unit in Edinburgh, with the greatest number of cases in one year

[1]   Fitzpatrick, M. (2001) *The Tyranny of Health: Doctors and the Regulation of Lifestyle*

[2]   See, for example, 'Vegetarian, 24, gets CJD', *Independent*, 22 August 1997; 'Family's anger as "vegetarian" dies of CJD', *The Times* (London), 28 April 2003

[3]   BSE and CJD Update, Parliamentary Office of Science and Technology, October 1997

being 28 in 2000. Even then, a third of those cases have not actually been confirmed by neuropathological examination. For the period 2008–10, just seven deaths have been reported. As a comparison, there have been 1,157 deaths from the long-standing 'sporadic' form of CJD – the disease almost no one had ever heard of before BSE – since 1990, amounting to roughly 55 deaths per year on average.

Researchers involved in the field are still worried that an epidemic may follow based on the long incubation periods of other prion diseases. However, even they must wonder why the trickle of cases 10 years ago has turned into a drip not a flood.

Others are less sympathetic to the mainstream explanation for vCJD. George Venters, a Scottish consultant in public health medicine, wrote a paper for the *British Medical Journal* in 2001 arguing that the epidemiological evidence showed there was no food-borne infection. If there really had been a food-based illness, the numbers affected would have started to rise sharply rather than falling away. Moreover, Venters was critical of the apparently limited effort to prove that vCJD was a truly novel disease and not simply a rare, but pre-existing condition. Despite the fact that pretty much the entire UK population would have been exposed to this infected meat, the numbers affected by the disease have been small and falling.

But the direct impact of vCJD has been the least important consequence of the panic. The significance of mad cow disease was in providing the moment where the government admitted to having got its advice to the public wrong. This has resulted in a lingering bad faith amongst the public in government announcements about food safety. More importantly, the government believes it is no longer trusted, and ever since has taken an almost insanely precautionary approach to food scares. Even though the vCJD epidemic had been hyped out of all proportion, the lesson that has been learned is that you can never be too careful, especially when it comes to making alterations to our food supply.

Frankenstein food: The GM panic

Perhaps the biggest effect of the BSE panic — at least in Europe — has been on the discussion of genetically modified (GM) foods. Between green groups demanding a precautionary approach to this 'tinkering with nature' and a general mistrust of any government assurance that food is safe, the result has been to shun this potentially invaluable technology.

It should be noted that all the plants and animals that we eat have already been genetically modified, in the sense that over the course of many years farmers have selected plants with a variety of desirable attributes and, by selective breeding, produced more productive versions. The history of agriculture is, in many ways, the history of such crop development. Nor has this process been a simple, painstaking business of cross-breeding. For example, for the past 80 years, in order to speed up the creation of new varieties, seeds have been exposed to radiation in order to increase the rate of mutation and provide a larger pool of genetic variations from which to select these desirable characteristics.

The controversial modern process known as genetic modification (or more precisely, transgenesis) takes this process further, by manipulating sections of DNA directly, and copying desirable attributes from entirely different species. For example, if wheat were found to be susceptible to a fungal infection and a variety of grass was found that was resistant to that infection, it would make sense to try to combine that resistance into wheat without losing any of the other positive characteristics of the wheat plant. This can be done using a combination of long-standing techniques but, in theory, transgenetic techniques should be quicker and more exact.

Transgenetic techniques remain very much in their infancy: nonetheless, the limited number of GM crops produced to date have generally been successful and popular with farmers. Studies and trials of GM crops, and the experience of their introduction across the world, have consistently failed to show that the crops pose any dangers for human health. Nor have the crops been shown to have a significant impact on the wider natural environment.

The first commercially available GM food was the FlavrSavr tomato, which was designed to have a longer shelf-life than regular tomatoes. Released in 1994, it was well accepted by US consumers, but it was simply not as profitable as other tomatoes produced by conventional methods. A version of this tomato was sold as tomato puree in Europe in 1996 as a marketing experiment without objection from consumers. But when researcher Árpád Puzstai suggested that a variety of genetically modified potato could cause intestinal damage (a claim dismissed by a later Royal Society report[4]), this gave campaigners the ammunition they needed to get GM foods withdrawn from supermarkets.

For the most part, however, there are only two kinds of trait produced by transgenetic methods that have been planted on a large scale. The first is herbicide-resistance, enabling farmers to spray crops with a herbicide — usually a glysophate-based product like Monsanto's Roundup — which only kills the weeds, not the crops. The other kind encourages the production of a bacterium — *Bacillus thuringiensis*, or Bt — which is poisonous to many common pests. For example, Bt-cotton is resistant to bollworms (moth larvae) that burrow into the plants. Bt-containing sprays have been used for decades, but adding the Bt-trait at the DNA level means that the insecticidal property is right there in the plant.

In the US, the authorities have taken a fairly *laissez-faire* attitude to GM foods. The plant in question is deemed not to be significantly different from existing plants unless a new toxin, nutrient or allergenic protein has been produced. For a while, a similar approach in Europe seemed likely, but Europe has been much more heavily influenced by precautionary thinking in relation to GM. As things currently stand, billions of acres around the world have been planted with GM crops; but in Europe any food with more than 0.9 per cent GM content must be labelled as such and super-

---

[4]   GM food study was 'flawed', BBC News, 18May 1999

markets have competed on the degree to which their goods are GM-free.

Why haven't Europeans been more keen to reap the benefits of these high-tech crops? The food policy writer and academic Robert Paarlberg makes an interesting point about consumer acceptance of GM foods:

> Consumers find it easy to reject GMO foods and crops because, so far, they have provided almost no direct consumer benefit. Genetically modified soybeans or corn do not taste better, look better, prepare better, or nourish better than conventional soybeans or corn. They are not noticeably cheaper because most of the economic gains from using the technology are captured by the farmer (who saves money by using less insecticide or fewer herbicides) or by the patent-owning biotechnology company. In the absence of any new consumer benefit, citizens in rich countries (few of whom are farmers) typically have little to lose when they reject agricultural GMOs.[5]

While Western consumers can afford to be ambivalent about GM, farmers and consumers in the developing world face a much more difficult choice. In 2002, during a serious food shortage, Zambia rejected aid from the US that contained GM food. This was partly because anti-GM campaigners had influenced the government, but also because there were fears that if GM seeds contaminated non-GM crops then Europe would never accept Zambian exports in the future. As Paalberg notes, attitudes to GM in the developing world depend on which market the country in question relates to: producers whose main market is North America are much more likely to embrace GM than countries that sell predominantly to Europe.

It should also be noted that the leading GM companies have done themselves few favours in this food-fearing climate. They have tended to overhype the benefits of the technology; in fact, only the simplest traits that have the greatest potential for commercial exploitation have been well developed so far, because the technology has proved to be trickier to utilise than expected. Transgenic methods seem to have been used as much because the resultant varieties have been

---

[5]   Paarlberg, R. (2010) *Food Politics: What Everyone Needs to Know*

easier to patent than those produced by other methods. And GM companies have done little to win the battle for the hearts and minds of the public, tending to come across as arrogant and monopolistic rather than endeavouring to provide something of benefit to consumers.

Every GM crop (or even genetically modified fish or animal) should be assessed for safety before coming to market, but near-blanket bans on new foods are simply irrational and will only hold back a valuable technology. And when countries from the USA to India and Brazil have utilised GM, we do have to ask how long Europe will be able to afford its po-faced commitment to lagging behind.

BSE and GM foods are only two of the epidemic of food panics that have afflicted the UK in recent years. Let's look at a few of the more mundane scares that grip the media and public imagination.

Heart attack on a plate

An influential food panic has grown out of the notion that eating too much fat—or more specifically, too much saturated fat—will lead to a heart attack. Saturated fats are usually associated with animal products like dairy products and meat, although some plant products like coconut oil actually contain more saturated fat. That's why the great British breakfast, once the calorie-rich and nutritious start to a day's work, is now seen as a 'heart attack on a plate'.

Advice on the NHS website makes clear the official advice:

> Saturated fat can raise our blood cholesterol over time, and so increase the risk of heart disease. It's the fat that most of us need to cut down on and is usually found in the following foods:
>
> - fatty cuts of meat
> - meat products including sausages and pies
> - butter, ghee and lard
> - cheese, especially hard cheese
> - cream, soured cream and ice cream
> - some savoury snacks and some sweets and chocolate
> - biscuits, cakes and pastries.

The idea is that excessive consumption of saturated fat leads to increased levels of blood cholesterol and this, in turn, causes heart disease. For an idea that is now assumed to be common sense, it only emerged after the Second World War. The tale of how the fat-cholesterol hypothesis went from ugly duckling to beautiful swan is neatly laid out by US science writer Gary Taubes in his book *Good Calories, Bad Calories*.

The theory that heart disease is caused by having too much cholesterol in our blood was devised and furiously promoted by Ancel Keys, a physiologist from the University of Minnesota, who first achieved fame by developing packs of mostly dry food for soldiers during the Second World War known as 'K-rations'. Some researchers initially believed that high levels of blood cholesterol were caused by simply consuming too much cholesterol itself. However, it quickly became apparent that the amount of cholesterol we eat has next to no impact on our cholesterol readings.

During a trip to Italy after the war, it was pointed out to Keys that while heart disease was an apparently increasing problem in the Western world, this was not the case in Naples. After travelling to the city with his wife, a medical technician familiar with the new procedure for measuring cholesterol, Keys concluded that it was the diet of the ordinary Neapolitan—containing very little meat—that was the key. Rich people ate more fat than the poor and were also more likely to develop heart disease.

Keys drew together further observations over subsequent years that reinforced his feeling that the consumption of fat led to higher cholesterol levels in the blood, which in turn led to atherosclerosis—ie, 'furry' arteries. At first, his peers were unconvinced. For example, in 1953 Keys had presented an analysis of six countries, which he said confirmed his thesis that heart disease rates and fat intake were closely related. However, when data from all the 22 countries where figures for diet and heart disease were available were taken together, Keys' association between fat and heart disease disappeared.

While the level of saturated fat in the diet does seem to be related to cholesterol in the blood, it is not at all clear that cholesterol is the villain that Keys painted it to be. A study as early as 1936 on New Yorkers who had met a violent death, as opposed to dying from a medical condition, found that cholesterol in these patients bore no relationship to the level of atherosclerosis that was found in autopsy.

The fat-and-heart-disease theory should have been laid to rest by a number of big research projects that reported in the early 1980s, most particularly the Multiple Risk Factor Intervention Trial (MRFIT), which encouraged a large number of middle-aged American men with high cholesterol to change their diet so as to reduce their saturated-fat intake and, therefore, their cholesterol. These test subjects were also encouraged to quit smoking and to treat their high blood pressure. Meanwhile, another large group of middle-aged men were left to their own devices. The result? Slightly more men in the low-fat diet group died than in the control group, but to all intents and purposes the results were the same.

Given that the low-fat group were also the ones getting help to quit smoking, the death rate for them should have been lower — even if their diet had no effect. As it was, the effects of other lifestyle changes seemed to be cancelled out by the very low-fat diet we are all still told to eat.

Another way to examine the problem would be to look at the effects of cholesterol-reducing drugs called statins. These have achieved something of a 'wonder drug' status in recent because of their effectiveness in reducing cholesterol levels. But do they prevent heart disease? A major review of the evidence published in 2011 found 'limited evidence' that giving statins to patients without heart disease would be cost effective and improve patient quality of life. While overall mortality did fall, the researchers expressed scepticism about whether the small improvements might be better explained by drug companies cherry-picking results

than any significant benefit from the drugs.[6] Can cholesterol really be the cause of heart disease if reducing it has so
little effect?

Given the failure to produce convincing evidence for the
cholesterol theory, how has the idea of measuring and low-
ering our cholesterol—most notably by avoiding fatty
foods—managed to maintain such an iron grip on the imagination of doctors and health advisers? Taubes notes a variety of key events, in particular the issuing of a number of
key reports in the 1960s and 1970s, which gave the official
stamp of approval to the cholesterol theory. Once a consensus had been established, contradictory ideas were frowned
upon or, more likely, simply ignored.

Taubes argues that we should in fact be aiming to eat a
low-carbohydrate diet, not a low-fat diet; and that, ironically, it is the advice to eat less fat—which means we eat
more carbohydrate to compensate—that is actually causing
heart disease (and obesity, for that matter). Whether or not
we should all switch to eating an Atkins-style diet is one
thing; but Taubes—and other critics like James Le Fanu and
Uffe Ravnskov—makes a convincing case for why the
obsession with cholesterol, and avoiding animal foods, is
misplaced.

A pinch of salt

Too much salt in our diet, we are told, increases blood pressure and this high blood pressure in turn increases the risk
of a heart attack or stroke. Just like the fat-causes-heart-
disease hypothesis, the idea that we need to cut our salt
intakes is treated entirely as common sense. The UK group
Consensus Action on Salt and Health (CASH) argues:

> A large number of studies have been conducted, *all of which*
> support the concept that salt intake is the major factor
> increasing population blood pressure. The diversity and
> strength of the evidence is much greater than for other life-
> style factors—eg, weight reduction, lack of fruit and vege-
> table consumption, and lack of exercise. The evidence that

[6]   Taylor, F. *et al.* (2011) Statins for the primary prevention of
         cardiovascular disease, Cochrane Library

links salt to blood pressure is as strong as that linking cigarette smoking to cancer and heart disease.[7] [My emphasis]

Yet this is simply not true. In fact, the evidence on salt and
blood pressure is downright contradictory. Tinkering
around with the amount of salt that we consume probably
won't do us much good, may actually be bad for us, and will
almost certainly make our food taste worse.

Sodium is absolutely crucial to flavouring food. Salt is
also one of the primary factors in flavour. Our tongues are
currently only believed to detect five tastes: sweet, sour, bitter, salt and umami (a fifth taste, discovered in the early
twentieth century, which is basically 'savouriness'). Making salt central to how we experience food almost certainly
evolved as a result of its importance to our health. As the
doyen of British cookery, Delia Smith, notes in her *Complete
Cookery Course*: 'It's amazing the difference salt makes to
food, almost magically bringing out the flavour of a soup or
sauce that may have seemed quite bland.'

In another cookery classic, *On Food and Cooking: The Science and Lore of the Kitchen*, Harold McGee reminds us how
salt has always been regarded as extremely valuable. It was
prescribed as an offering to God in the Old Testament. In the
book of Ezekiel (16.4), there is reference to the custom of
rubbing salt on newborns. Roman soldiers were paid a special allowance — a salarium — to buy the stuff (the source of
the word 'salary'). The control of salt, and revolts against
such control, have been influential from the French Revolution to Gandhi's India. Even Jesus knew the importance of
the white stuff, describing believers as the 'salt of the earth'.

As for health, it is striking that in almost all countries
where salt is freely available, more salt is consumed than
the guideline amount suggested by CASH and the UK's
health authorities of six grammes per day for adults. (The
World Health Organisation has suggested an even lower
target of five grammes per day.) In Japan, with a famously
high life expectancy, salt consumption is roughly double
the UK target.

[7]   Salt and blood pressure, Consensus Action on Salt and Health
       http://bit.ly/gmxzcD

Nor is it the case that encouraging population-wide reduction in salt intake is necessarily a good idea. A review in the *British Medical Journal* in 2002 concluded:

> Intensive interventions, unsuited to primary care or population prevention programmes, provide only small reductions in blood pressure and sodium excretion, and effects on deaths and cardiovascular events are unclear. Advice to reduce sodium intake may help people on antihypertensive drugs to stop their medication while maintaining good blood pressure control.[8]

In other words, if you already have high blood pressure, it may make sense to do everything you can to cut it, so cutting your salt intake might be worth a try. For the rest of us, such interventions are probably of little benefit.

What is remarkable about all of this is that the level of sodium in the cells in our bodies must be kept very tightly under control for a whole host of biological reasons. As a result, we have evolved over millions of years the ability to tune these sodium levels very finely. It's a sign of our bossy-boots times that official salt level targets are assumed to be more effective than our own exquisite homeostatic mechanisms.

Counting the costs of five-a-day

There is, apparently, no health problem that cannot be solved by eating more fruit and vegetables. Conversely, failing to eat five portions of fruit and veg a day could be causing ill health. Yet when long-term studies of such diets have been undertaken, they have failed to provide the evidence to back up the assumption that fruit and veg have such miraculous, health-giving properties.

The NHS website provides the official reasons for encouraging us to 'just eat more' [fruit and veg]:

> Fruit and vegetables taste delicious and there's so much variety to choose from; they're a good source of vitamins and minerals, including folate, vitamin C and potassium; they're an excellent source of dietary fibre, which helps

---

[8]   Hooper, L. *et al.* (2002) Systematic review of long term effects of advice to reduce

maintain a healthy gut and prevent constipation and other digestion problems and a diet high in fibre can also reduce your risk of bowel cancer; they can help reduce the risk of heart disease, stroke and some cancers.[9]

Many people may believe that fruit and veg taste nice, but is it really the place of the NHS to tell us this? Vitamins and minerals are a good idea, but there are plenty of other sources of these nutrients. For example, meat, dairy product and cereals like wheat are rich in nutrients. Just to complicate things, 'potatoes and cassava don't count because they mainly contribute starch to the diet', despite the fact they are both good sources of vitamin C. Yams are out, too. Plantains don't count, despite the fact that they are more nutritious in many ways than their close cousins, bananas.

Indeed, there are all sorts of other esoteric rules to be followed to meet your five-a-day target: only one portion of fruit juice counts, and only two portions of smoothies; only one portion of beans or pulses is allowed (they're not very nutritious, apparently); fruit and veg found in ready meals need to be treated with caution because you may find such foods contain a lot of salt and sugar.

What about all that lovely dietary fibre? A variety of studies have shown a weak association between dietary fibre and reductions in colorectal cancer but these associations are so weak that they are not generally statistically significant. In any event, epidemiological studies have to be treated very carefully as there are always confounding factors that could be influencing the outcome, so even a strong association would only be indicative of an effect — it wouldn't prove one.

Far better are randomised controlled trials that specifically test for the effect of fibre on health. An article by Lawlor and Ness in 2003 noted:

> To date there have been five randomised trials of dietary fibre in high-risk patients — those with a previous history of an adenomatous polyp but no previous history of cancer. None of these trials has found fibre to be effective at reduc-

---

[9]   Why 5 A Day? NHS Choices, Department of Health
      http://bit.ly/h1CjL7

ing the recurrence of polyps or the occurrence of colorectal cancer.

Perhaps fibre protects against heart disease instead. Yet, Lawlor and Ness write:

> [I]f fibre really is protective against heart disease and cancers (the two biggest killers in the Western world) then one would expect it to have an important impact on all-cause mortality. To date randomized trials have found no evidence that dietary fibre confers any short-term benefit on all-cause mortality. Indeed, a large study on British men post myocardial infarction suggested, if anything, that mortality was higher among those allocated to dietary advice aimed at increasing fibre consumption.[10]

In short, fibre in our diets won't help us live longer.

Maybe the effect of fruit and veg relates to other kinds of disease? A major study published in 2010 by Paulo Boffetta *et al.* suggests that the five-a-day advice has either very little or no effect on cancer in general. The study concludes that: 'A very small inverse association between intake of total fruits and vegetables and cancer risk was observed in this study'. But this finding was not statistically significant, which means to all intents and purposes there was no effect at all.[11]

A major study in America, the Women's Health Initiative Dietary Modification Trial, which published its results in 2006 and 2007, was a very large and expensive randomised controlled trial of the effect of diet and weight on breast cancer, colon cancer, heart disease and stroke amongst 49,000 women over an eight-year period. While the control group ate a typical American diet, the study group were encouraged to eat a low-fat, high-grain diet including that all-important five-a-day. Yet there were no statistically significant differences found between the two groups.

---

[10] Lawlor, D., Ness, A. (2003) Commentary: The rough world of nutritional epidemiology: Does dietary fibre prevent large bowel cancer?, *International Journal of Epidemiology*

[11] Boffetta, P. *et al.* (2010) Fruit and Vegetable Intake and Overall Cancer Risk in the European Prospective Investigation Into Cancer and Nutrition (EPIC), *Journal of the National Cancer Institute*

So if the big, gold-standard trials aren't providing the evidence for eating five-a-day, why bother? The NHS is telling us to eat at least 400 grammes (roughly one pound in weight) of fruit and veg every day, something that most people would find to be a chore. Indeed, UK government statistics for 2006 suggest that just 28 per cent of men and 32 per cent of women eat their 'five a day'. Are we really surprised by this?

Not only is there very limited support for eating five a day: according to Helen Rumbelow, writing in *The Times* (London) in 2010, the number involved was chosen for marketing reasons, not on the basis of scientific evidence. Marion Nestle, professor of nutrition at New York University, told *The Times* that the idea came from 'Susan Foerster, the head nutritionist in California', in 1988, who 'had the bright idea of promoting fruit and vegetable consumption in a state which was a big fruit and vegetable producer'. Tim Lang, professor of food policy at London's City University, tells Rumbelow:

> We all understand targets in the policy world. I remember being in the room when we were being briefed by Americans on five-a-day, which we adopted from them. They chose five partly as it was considered a nice round sum and partly because it seemed possible, given how low consumption of fruit and vegetables was.[12]

Paulo Boffetta is quoted as saying: 'We have to abandon this idea that there's something miraculous in diet. It's not true for fruit and vegetables as a whole, and even less true for fruit and vegetables individually.'

So what has been the effect of the five-a-day campaign? It does not seem to have got us to eat substantially more fruit and veg. Even if it had, it would not have any noticeable impact on our health. But perhaps it has had one impact: to increase the amount of food—and money—we waste. I cannot be alone in having bought an extra pack of apples or bananas on the basis that 'I should get more fruit', only to find the stuff rotting in the fridge or the fruit bowl a week or

---

[12] How the 'five a day' mantra was born, *The Times* (London), 13 April 2010 http://thetim.es/f1vDAq

two later. The alternative has been to eat that extra fruit and veg in some processed form — like a fruit smoothie — that lasts longer but costs a comparative fortune. No wonder that a company like smoothie makers Innocent — a relatively new player in the UK food market — has gone from nothing in 1999 to high-profile Coca-Cola takeover target in 2010. Kerching!

'Five-a-day' may not seem like a panic. It is, after all, a piece of advice about what we should eat. But the implication of that campaign has been to suggest that we will die younger than we need to if we don't start eating our fruit and veg. In reality, there has never been anything like sufficient evidence to back this claim up. The UK population has been subjected to the prejudices of policy wonks and health guardians for no good reason.

Meat and cancer

The flipside of the claim that fruit and veg are a panacea is the idea that red meat — particularly processed meat — is downright deadly. Yet the evidence is, again, flimsy.

The organisation that has pushed the meat-and-cancer link more than any other is the World Cancer Research Fund, which has aggressively pursued the idea that many cancers are caused by diet, lack of exercise and other environmental factors and are, therefore, preventable. In a press release in 2009, WCRF declares:

> There is convincing scientific evidence that eating processed meat increases bowel cancer risk and this is why WCRF recommends people avoid eating processed meat. In the UK, scientists estimate about 3,700 bowel cancer cases could be prevented if everyone ate less than 70g of processed meat a week, which is roughly the equivalent of three rashers of bacon.

Yet even according to the organisation's own surveys of the evidence, the link between colorectal (ie, bowel) cancer and processed meat is fairly weak, although 16 epidemiological studies do point to their being some effect. The key here is 'convincing evidence'. The studies in question suggest that the people who eat the most processed and red meat have an increased risk of somewhere between 15 per cent and 45 per cent. But given the crude nature of these studies – often based on a questionnaire of a whole variety of different eating and other personal habits in the first week of the study followed by checks on disease status some years later – there is room for all sorts of confounding factors to creep in. Are the kinds of people who eat a lot of processed meat different in other ways, too, like being poorer?

That's why the US National Cancer Institute declared in 1994 that 'in epidemiological research, [increases in risk of less than 100 per cent] are considered small and are usually difficult to interpret. Such increases may be due to chance, statistical bias, or the effects of confounding factors that are sometimes not evident'. In other words, if a particular factor does not at least double the risk of a particular disease or condition occurring, treat that result with a pinch of salt. The link between lung cancer and active smoking, for example, is unambiguous, with increases in risk more in the order of 2,000 per cent, not 15 per cent. In such circumstances, correlation seems a good indication of causation. The red/processed meat link to cancer is nothing like as strong.

However, as health writer Sandy Szwarc points out, WCRF failed to include some very good-quality studies that contradict this finding. For example, a study by Harvard University researchers, published in *Proceedings of the American Association of Cancer Research* in 2004, found that: 'Greater intake of either red meat (excluding processed meat) or processed meat was not related to colorectal cancer risk.'

Another study, from the US government's National Toxicology Program in 2001 found no link between sodium nitrite – the preservative salt in cooked meats that provides the distinctive pink colour – and cancer. That sodium nitrite is absolutely vital, however, in preventing diseases like botulism appearing in preserved meat. Szwarc also notes that the prevention of infection is important in preventing cancer, too.[13]

One other important lesson is this: the thing that should concern us is not relative risk but absolute risk. For example, if our lifetime risk of bowel cancer is five per cent and eating processed meat increases it to six per cent, that is a 20 per cent increase in the relative risk of developing bowel cancer. But in reality, it is a one-in-a-hundred increase in risk, which seems a lot smaller. Is that worth foregoing bacon for?

[13] What's the evidence cancers are our own fault? *Junkfood Science*, 1 November 2007 http://bit.ly/hz5OKD

Chapter Seven

Eating the planet

Back in 2006, I attended a Hay Festival event at London's Garrick Theatre called 'The Ethical Food Debate'. It wasn't much of a debate since all four speakers—and most of the seemingly well-to-do audience—were quite in agreement about the need to protect the environment, eat organic, avoid chemicals and reduce 'food miles'. But amid all the Henriettas, Rosies and Thomasinas, it was comments by panellist Ken Livingstone—then London mayor—that stuck in my mind.

Livingstone seemed rather overwhelmed (and ill-informed) about the environment and food. He claimed, in defence of organic food, that 'the smallest amount of artificial or toxic substances can cause all sorts of problems, not just cancers but everything else'. He then went on to assert that London's pollution problems had got worse rather than better in recent decades. 'I grew up in the postwar world where it was heavy, dirty old soot you could wash away—now it's particulates and nitrous oxoids [sic] which are just getting worse and worse', he stated, which apparently 'goes a long way to explaining the huge increase in kids in asthma and eczema and hay fever'.

If it wasn't the chemicals that would kill you, in Livingstone's mind at least, it would be the blazing heat of a rapidly-warming planet. Livingstone asserted that the 'tipping point for irreversible climate change is most probably four or five years away at most', which apparently means we need to crack down on agribusiness now, because agribusiness is a 'disproportionate' generator of carbon emissions and 'food miles'.

The upshot of Livingstone's nightmares about pesticides, global warming and pollution was that he found himself in a state of paralysis in front of the supermarket fruit and veg. Should he eat organic, or go for the veggies with the fewest food miles? Or maybe he should worry more about whether his purchases were Fairtrade or kind to the rainforest?

Livingstone's fears are all exaggerated, but his views seem typical of the kind of debate that happens more and more about food, health and the environment. There is a growing concern that wasteful, polluting industrial agriculture is killing us and murdering the planet.

Choking on our food

Since growing and distributing food is a major human activity, it is unsurprisingly a significant source of greenhouse gas emissions. These are generated in a variety of ways. At the farm, there are carbon dioxide emissions from using oil to drive machinery; nitrous oxide comes from the breaking down in the soil of fertiliser, which itself is usually made by combining hydrogen from natural gas (a fossil fuel) with nitrogen from the air; the farmyard animals will often eat grain grown elsewhere then belch out methane in great quantities. If land that was once pristine forest — whose trees would absorb carbon dioxide from the atmosphere — is cleared to grow crops or to graze cattle, the net effect is to increase greenhouse gases in the atmosphere. If the land is cleared by burning down the trees first, the effect is even worse.

When all this food is then harvested (or slaughtered), machinery is used in the process, then the food is transported possibly thousands of miles, requiring more oil to be burned both for locomotion and refrigeration. Much of it will then be processed in one way or another, becoming anything from ready meals to red wine. When it arrives at the supermarket, cars roll up to take small chunks of this total supply home, burning yet more fuel on the journey before the contents of the shopping bags are frozen or refrigerated. Finally, the food is cooked (assuming it hasn't already rotted through neglect), using yet more gas or electricity. Even if we don't eat food from the supermarket, we may still drive to a restaurant or takeaway to eat food cooked by someone else.

Thus, agriculture has a large 'carbon footprint'. The World Resources Institute estimates, based on 2005 data, that agriculture generated 13.8 per cent of the total greenhouse impact of human activity. However, this appears to count only emissions from the farm itself, so transportation, storage, cooking and deforestation would be important additional factors. In his book *Waste*, Tristram Stuart argues that eating actually accounts for 41 per cent of UK greenhouse gas emissions — but then adds that this may itself be an underestimate.

Given that eating is our most basic necessity, it is hardly surprising that it holds such a dominant place in the totality of human activity. Setting aside any scepticism about whether climate change is as serious as many environmentalists believe, the question is how much the emissions caused by food production and consumption present a problem — and what can be done about them.

A truck-load of food fears

One of the most popular ideas for dealing with emissions is to reduce transportation. If we eat as much as we can from relatively local sources, goes this thinking, then emissions will decline and warming will be slowed down. If food were labelled with the distance it had travelled, consumers could make informed ethical decisions about what they eat, bringing us back to Ken Livingstone's conundrum. Hence, the idea of 'food miles'.

It's such a simple concept: in order to understand the environmental impact of the food we eat, we should take into account how far it travels 'from fork to fork' — from digging up the soil to digging into our dinner. The idea has been picked up by everyone from ethical advisers to multi-nationals.

The term 'food miles' was coined in the 1990s by Professor Tim Lang, currently at City University in London but also a veteran of numerous institutions and organisations that have fretted about our food, from the London Food Commission (formed when Ken Livingstone first ran the capital in his 'loony leftie' era in the 1980s) to the campaign group, Sustain. For Lang, 'The idea behind food miles — or food kilometres, as they should probably now be known — was and remains simple. We wanted people to think about where their food came from, to reinject a cultural dimension into arcane environmental debates about biodiversity in farms.' What that means for consumers, says Lang, is that wherever possible they should 'shop locally and buy local produce'.[1]

Following Lang's creation of the 'food miles' idea, we have been inundated with shocked articles and campaigns raising awareness about the distances involved in bringing together a plate of food. In the UK, we get beef from Argentina (6,700 miles), pineapples from Ghana (3,100 miles), tomatoes from Spain (800 miles) or even Saudi Arabia (3,100 miles), prawns from Indonesia (7,300 miles) and lamb from New Zealand (11,700 miles). Put together a typical plate of NZ lamb, potatoes from Israel (2,200 miles), green beans from Zambia (4,900 miles) and wash it down with a fruity Shiraz from Australia (9,000 miles) and your one course with plonk has collectively journeyed 27,800 miles. Gulp.

Ever keen to do the right thing, supermarkets started slapping 'airplane' stickers on to their produce to indicate when food had been flown in or travelled a long way. The British agriculture periodical *Farmers Weekly* ran a campaign in 2006, declaring: 'Local food is miles better'. According to the 'campaign facts' page, food miles 'hurt the environment', 'reduce freshness', 'mean less security' (from those unstable countries we have to buy food from now),

[1]   Origin unknown, *Guardian*, 3 August 2005

and make it harder to 'monitor production and welfare standards'.

The trouble with the concept of food miles is that it is not only simple: it is simple-minded. It even caused a little cat-fight in the green movement, when outraged members of New Zealand's Green Party wrote to their British counterparts to protest at the eco-calumny that we shouldn't buy Kiwi food. 'The total greenhouse emissions released in the production and transport of dairy and lamb shipped to Britain from New Zealand are lower than the emissions generated by the production of dairy and lamb in Britain', declared New Zealand Green Party co-leader, Russel Norman.

Norman pointed to research from New Zealand's Lincoln University showing that simply counting the miles travelled was little help in assessing the 'ecological footprint' of a particular foodstuff. For example, lamb reared on sunny New Zealand pasture and then shipped halfway round the world to the UK creates fewer carbon emissions than meat from animals reared on the rather less luscious grass in the fields of Wales or Scotland, because UK farmers have to add extra feed to the diets of their animals, which is grown using fertilisers and then transported to the farm—all of which emits carbon dioxide. There are lots of other examples—like Spanish tomatoes—where growing food in sunnier climes and then shipping it to Britain uses far fewer resources and emits less pollution than growing crops in less favourable circumstances closer to home.

Even the dreaded green bean air-freighted from Kenya, which has become the *bête noire* of foodies, cannot be so neatly cast as a villain. Professor Gareth Edwards-Jones, an expert on African agriculture, told the *Observer* in 2008:

> Beans there are grown using manual labour—nothing is mechanised. They don't use tractors, they use cow muck as fertiliser; and they have low-tech irrigation systems in Kenya. They also provide employment to many people in the developing world. So you have to weigh that against the air miles used to get them to the supermarket.[2]

[2]   How the myth of food miles hurts the planet, *Observer*, 23 March 2008

The *Observer* also quoted Dr Adrian Williams of the National Resources Management Centre at Cranfield University: 'The concept of food miles is unhelpful and stupid. It doesn't inform about anything except the distance travelled'. It seems that there are so many different factors that go into the production, transportation, processing, selling, purchasing and cooking of all foods that any exercise in assessing ecological impact will only serve to provide gainful employment for environmental impact bean-counters.

Aside from the sheer folly of the exercise, assessing our food in terms of its ecological impact is really a campaigning point, a condemnation of the world market in food and of industrialised food production. Lang himself would no doubt argue that the notion of food miles is aimed at getting us to think, rather than capturing all of the environmental side effects associated with food. However, if we are going to think hard about where our food comes from, we should also think hard about where the concept of food miles comes from. The real target is the modernisation and globalisation of food. But these two trends have provided us with both a far greater range of different food products than our grandparents would have known, meaning our diets are more interesting, and it has made food much cheaper, allowing more and more people to eat well and to devote their hard-earned cash to other things instead.

If the notion of 'food miles' is supposed to put us off modernising agriculture and taking advantage of a global division of labour, then it is a very bad idea.

Local food for local people

The perversity of the demand for local food was made clear to me during a debate I took part in at London's Real Food Festival in 2008. *Ecologist* publisher and then Conservative Party environment adviser Zac Goldsmith (now a Conservative MP), told the gathered audience that local food was crucial—perhaps an even more important issue for green foodies than organic food. But when a member of the audience who lived in inner-city London asked the panel how she could eat 'local' food, Goldsmith was a bit stuck. It depends, said the billionaire's son, offering that 'local' might mean the Caribbean if you were talking about bananas. So, 'local' could mean 4,500 miles away?

Critics of modern food production seem to want to stop the world and get off — no more so than so-called 'locavores', who aim to eat only eat food produced in close proximity to their homes. This promotes a kind of ethically-sound parochialism, where we are asked to spurn the cornucopia of world agriculture for a narrow and puritan diet based on the produce of Farmer Giles down the road. (And in these days of right-on gentlemen farmers, Giles is more likely to be his first name than his surname.)

The trend to food globalisation and specialisation has been a very good thing. Rising productivity means that workers in the developed world are freed from the grind of providing the essentials of life and can go and do something less boring instead. Perversely, just when this globalisation of food supply looks like it might be on the road to getting rid of scarcity, food campaigners seem to want to drag us back to the dreary diets of the past and make us pay more for the privilege. Meanwhile, those African farmers desperate for more hi-tech, profit-turning agricultural methods are patronisingly presented as (literally) down-to-earth models for Western consumer society — indicating just how little the 'grow local' foodies understand about the back-breaking reality of subsistence farming.

The beef with meat

In an interview with me in 2009, animal rights philosopher Peter Singer put the green case against eating meat:

> I believe that if we aim to get to a sustainable place in terms of greenhouse gas emissions, it's going to be very hard to have large herds of cattle and sheep as we do at present. That problem, combined with opposition to factory farming, really does mean we have to move towards vegetarian and even vegan diets in the medium term.[3]

---

[3]   It's time to stop exploiting animals for food, *spiked*, 14 September 2009

Singer's view has been widely supported by leading figures in the debate about climate change. 'In terms of immediacy of action and the feasibility of bringing about [emission] reductions in a short period of time, [avoiding meat] clearly is the most attractive opportunity', said the head of the Intergovernmental Panel on Climate Change, Rajendra Pachauri in 2008, further suggesting that we 'Give up meat for one day [a week] initially and decrease it from there.'[4] Pachauri, himself a vegetarian, apparently had the scientific backing of the UN Food and Agriculture Organisation (FAO), which produced a report in 2006 — *Livestock's Long Shadow* — claiming that 18 per cent of global greenhouse gas emissions were due to producing food from animals. That is even greater than the level of emissions produced by transport. Forget all those carbon-spewing cars, we were told, it's our taste for burgers and chicken that was really to blame for screwing up the planet.

Perhaps surprisingly, the best critique of the idea that eating meat is wrecking the planet has come from a dyed-in-the-wool environmentalist who was, for a while, the co-editor of the *Ecologist* magazine. In *Meat: A Benign Extravagance*, Simon Fairlie has crunched the numbers on the impact of meat and concludes that those greens who have condemned meat as inherently problematic are wrong. One of the many jobs Fairlie has done over the years was as a stockman in a communally-run farm he refers to as 'Happy Valley'. The group's diet was essentially vegetarian, so it refused to use the products from the farm's animals, yet still imported certain specific high-fat or high-protein foods from around the world. Fairlie notes, a little despairingly:

> In short, Happy Valley was producing, from the grass that we all walked on, a substantial proportion of the protein and fat that we required for our nutrition, but we weren't eating it and instead were importing it from countries where people go hungry.[5]

[4] UN says eat less meat to curb global warming, *Guardian*, 7 September 2008

[5] A benign extravagance? *Permaculture* no. 65, Autumn 2010

In 2004, Fairlie left the group, citing its attitude to meat as a contributory factor to his decision. With his curiosity sparked by the debates he had been having, he set out to investigate the ecological impact of meat.

Long before that FAO report in 2006, vegetarians and vegans had argued that meat is a very wasteful use of land. As Fairlie shows, there is some truth in the idea that you get more food from growing crops than producing meat. For example, producing one kilo of beef really does seem to take about 10 kilos of feed, though the figure is lower for pork and chicken. The implication that many people draw from that bald statement is that we could feed 10 times more people if we switched all land used for meat production over to growing grain.

But, once again, life is just not that simple. Animals fed on grass are often occupying land that is unsuitable for growing crops: they take a low-value source of energy and protein — grass — and turn it into high-value foods like meat and milk. Suddenly, that ratio of 10:1 starts to change according to the degree to which animals are the only way of deriving food in particular circumstances, whether it is sheep on a Welsh hillside or goats in arid desert-like conditions. Pigs cannot eat grass, but they'll eat just about anything else, so they can be an extremely useful means of recycling organic material that we can't eat, including human food waste and the bits of crops that we don't eat.

We should also bear in mind that animals provide products and services beyond food that would have to be replaced if we did not use them for meat, milk, eggs and so on. In some cases food is the by-product of animal production, not the main purpose. The products include leather from the hides of cattle and goats, gelatine from bones, and wool from sheep. Even when meat or milk is the main reason for rearing animals, little of the animal is wasted. Meat processors often boast that they use everything but the oink, moo or baa.

Less obvious to ignorant townies (like me) are the services provided by animals. Fairlie makes the point that animals are not simply consumers of the soil's fertility, but

transporters of it, too. If you have sheep on a mixed-produc-
tion farm, for example, you can have them graze relatively
poor-quality land during the day, then keep them at night in
a field that will be used for crops. Our little woolly friends
will excrete fertility into the field, free of charge.

Animal foods also provide important variety in our diets.
We don't just eat high-productivity vegetable foods like
wheat and potatoes. We also need – and want – to eat other
foods from salad vegetables to legumes that are simply
much less productive in terms of the sheer quantity of
nutrition they provide. Eating some animal products –
especially in circumstances where crops cannot be grown
– makes a great deal of sense even if, overall, it is a little
less efficient than the most productive plants.

On the question of emissions, Fairlie is critical of the UN
food report *Livestock's Long Shadow*, which, he argues, was
written to bolster the case for intensive meat production
(that is, keeping cattle in giant sheds and feeding them
grain) against extensive production (for example, putting
more and more land over to pasture). A significant proportion of the emissions attributed by the report to meat production, for example, is actually due to the clearing of
Amazon rainforest. But as Fairlie notes, this tree-felling has
slowed sharply in recent years, and animals are often simply an excuse to occupy land and keep it clear. The land grab
is the primary thing; the farming of animals is just a
by-product.

Another third of emissions comes from the use of fertilisers to grow feed crops for animals. But if we didn't produce
meat, we'd still need to eat, so some of those emissions
would occur in the process of producing plant foods
instead. Furthermore, if the kind of terrain that can currently only produce food by farming animals was left
undisturbed, then wild animals would move in to replace
domesticated ones – with all the farting, belching and defe-
cation associated with those beasts, too. One study that
Fairlie quotes suggests that in 1500, the huge herds of bison
that occupied the relatively untouched landscape of North

America would have generated three million tonnes of methane per year.

Fairlie's conclusion is that if we stopped devoting large areas of agricultural land to growing crops simply to feed to animals and only produced meat from pasture, from waste food, or from animals like chickens that are relatively good converters of grain to meat and eggs, then we could enjoy animal foods with relatively little additional impact on the environment compared to going vegetarian.

Fairlie's work has been warmly welcomed by a variety of environmental commentators, even some whom Fairlie roundly attacks in his book. In a sense, this isn't surprising. Fairlie's analysis squares an awkward circle for these carbon-counters, making the idea of accepting personal responsibility for greenhouse gas emissions more palatable for the wider public. The message is: you are screwing up the planet but if you eat less meat, or the right kind, you'll be making a major difference without having to become some dull, anaemic vegan.

While *Meat* provides plenty of ammunition to use against the tofu-munching set, Fairlie's outlook remains informed by the idea that humanity is a consumer of finite resources and a polluter of the atmosphere: he even refers in passing to 'overdeveloped countries'. Thus, in Fairlie's view, meat is actually less of a threat to the environment than many think, but only the right kind of meat: more pigs, more grass feeding, and definitely none of those nasty (but very efficient) feedlots that fatten thousands of cattle up on grain. In the obsession with greenhouse gas emissions, the fact — so unapologetically stated by Delia Smith[6] — that hundreds of millions of people enjoy cheaper meat as a result of the industrialisation of these processes is ignored.

Reducing our waste lines

If avoiding food miles and meat don't, after all, make much difference to the fate of the planet, avoiding waste might

[6]   Delia Smith: 'Battery chickens are necessary to feed poor families', *Daily Mail*, 15 February 2008

seem a better bet. In his book, *Waste*, Tristram Stuart argues that we could greatly reduce the environmental impact of eating if we simply ate the vast majority of what was grown. At every stage of the process from field to factory and from supermarket to dinner table, we manage to waste a considerable proportion of eatable food. Some of this is unavoidable, of course. But what is really alarming is how much good food is wasted that could be eaten if the best practices were followed.

For example, the weekly shop from the modern, Western supermarket has had some enormous benefits in terms of convenience, cost and the range and quality of food available to the vast majority of the population. However, it does open up the possibility of food waste. When food was bought no more than a day or so before it was used, and when household budgets were too tight to allow much waste, the vast majority of food purchased was eaten. Now, with consumers making educated guesses about what might be needed for the week, poor purchasing (and poorer fridge management) can mean that more food ends up in the bin. The UK Waste and Resources Action Programme (WRAP) claims that households dispose of 8.3million tonnes of food each year.

To some extent, this is a nice problem to have: it's partly a product of food being cheap. Food and non-alcoholic drinks made up 21 per cent of household expenditure in 1971, falling to 12 per cent in 1991 and just nine per cent in 2005/06, according to the UK Office for National Statistics. For low-income households, the proportion is higher, but for most people the single most important item of living costs now consumes just a tenth of our incomes. We can afford to be fickle about what we eat and disorganised with our purchasing.

The problem is compounded by the confusion around date labelling: there are labels for 'use-by', 'sell-by' and 'best before' date, all with quite different meanings. But for many of us, if the food in the fridge has passed that date, it gets chucked regardless of whether it seems useable or not. In reality, only the 'use-by' date is making any statement about the safety of food, and even then it is usually extremely conservative. As Lord Haskins, former boss of food manufacturing giant Northern Foods, tells Stuart, many of these label dates are 'excessive, over-reactive and absurdly unnecessary ... manufacturers assume everyone is an idiot; and on the other hand, the public are very stupid to take these dates seriously'.

There are other ways in which we waste food thanks to supermarket practices. For example, buy-one-get-one-free offers (or BOGOFs, as they are known in the trade) can be a recipe for waste when it comes to perishable foods — unless, of course, you can quickly get through two packs of the fruit or veg in question before it goes off. Combined with the relentless lectures to eat more fruit and veg, shoppers stock up on food that they will barely touch. The result is not a population fizzing with vitamin goodness but fruit bowls that look like diseased still-lifes, as one half of that two-for-one deal quietly rots. The obsession with health has done little to make us healthier, but fear of missing vital nutrients seems to have added to the amount we waste.

Further along the food chain, supermarkets are also big wasters of food. Stuart estimates that the seven biggest food retailers in the UK waste 367,000 tonnes of food per year. Much of this is fit to eat, as Stuart's years of experience living off the contents of supermarket bins as a so-called 'freegan' demonstrate. That said, a little perspective on that figure is required. Given that most food for the 60 million people in the UK comes from those big retailers, that amounts to just six kilogrammes of food per person per year — or about 16 grammes (just over half an ounce) per day. That actually sounds pretty efficient. And, as Stuart admits, smaller shops often throw away a much bigger proportion of their stock.

To this can be added the food wasted in other branches of retail, such as sandwich shops. As Stuart describes, it often makes more sense economically to over-produce food so that customers can buy right up to the end of the day than run out of stock and risk missing out on a sale. That's because the selling price of ready-to-eat food is often two or three times the cost of the ingredients.

A few years ago, I was a member of the jury in a drugs case at Southwark Crown Court in London. The accused, a young, homeless Polish man, had been arrested with a quantity of ecstasy tablets that seemed a few too many to be for personal use. He claimed he had just received them as payment for doing some work for a friend. The prosecuting barrister was unconvinced by his story. Given how poor he was, surely he would want payment in cash so that he could buy food? The defendant looked puzzled. Why, he asked, would he need money for food when he could eat the food left in the rubbish bags behind sandwich shops? The barrister was clearly unacquainted with either freeganism or the survival strategies of the modern London homeless.

However, freeganism only applies to what happens at the back of the store. Supermarkets are also responsible for a great deal of waste by farmers and food manufacturers. One area of particular concern is the need to meet cosmetic standards. British growers are subject to European regulations on the size and appearance of fruit and vegetables: so, as Stuart points out, carrots less than one centimetre in diameter cannot be sold. But the standards demanded by the supermarkets are almost invariably stricter and more infuriating than those laid down by the European Commission. If a cucumber isn't quite straight enough, or a carrot not orange enough, it can be rejected. In his book, Stuart talks to one farmer, Guy Poskitt, who typically has 25–30 per cent of his carrots 'out-graded' by the buyers at Wal-Mart's UK subsidiary, Asda. The standards of more upmarket stores, like Marks and Spencer, are even higher.

Things get even trickier because supermarkets impose onerous contracts on farmers to supply specific amounts of fruit and veg at particular times. If the farmer cannot deliver the full amount, he risks losing his contract. The result is that farmers over-plant and, even then, may still have to buy from other farmers to meet the terms of their contract if their own fields don't produce as much of a crop as expected.

Similar problems arise for food manufacturers thanks to the ordering practices of the supermarkets. One example Stuart offers is in relation to sandwiches, where producers often have little more than 24 hours notice of the size of a particular order. They need to be prepared for the full agreed quantity of, say, bacon and tomato sandwiches but if the supermarkets decide they don't need so many, the short notice is often too late to prevent the ordering in of perishable supplies. Worse, supermarkets are extremely sensitive to the idea that excess product bearing their brand will end up elsewhere. The result is that sandwiches that don't go to the store get binned.

However, it is wrong to be overly pessimistic about waste, which is a normal by-product of buying and selling on the market. Producers and retailers can, after all, only make educated guesses as to what will sell at any particular time and so there will almost always be some goods left over that cannot be sold, no matter how cleverly products are ordered in and surplus goods are discounted. Wherever there is choice and people can afford to be choosy, there will be waste. It is, of course, preferable to reduce waste to a minimum. But the existence of waste is actually a sign of social progress.

The problem of food waste is by no means exclusive to the developed world. In fact, food losses in developing countries are likely to have a far bigger impact on people who spend 50 per cent or more of their income on food than on those in the developed world who spend less than 10 per cent. This is particularly true for post-harvest losses. For example, storage facilities for crop surpluses are often poor; refrigeration and other preservation techniques are often unavailable; pests may attack food both in the field and after harvest. The agronomist Vaclav Smil has estimated that if all low-income countries were to lose 15 per cent of their annual crop of grain, that would amount to 150million tonnes of cereals — six times the additional amount required to turn the deficient diets of the world's malnourished people into adequate ones. Losses of just four per cent should be possible.

In other words, we could in theory feed the world just by wasting less food.

Stuart argues, along with many others, that food waste in the developed world snatches food from the mouths of the hungry elsewhere. Resources that should be used to feed the poor are diverted to satisfy the wasteful desires of the rich. Yet this suggests a considerable degree of economic illiteracy. Food supply flows from economic demand, not from human need. If the West didn't waste so much food, the result is more likely to be a reduction in the amount of food produced, not a decline in malnutrition.

Nor is it the case that we are wasting land in the West by growing food that is only thrown away. In fact, a trend in recent years has been for the retirement of land from production. As the writer James Heartfield notes: 'For more than 20 years now, both the US and the European Union have pursued policies designed to reduce food output. They have introduced policies that reward farmers for retiring land from production (such as the EU's set-aside and wilderness schemes)'. He continues:

> The programmes of land retirement and reservation have been so successful worldwide that between 1982 and 2003, national parks grew from nine million square kilometres to 19 million, 12.5 per cent of the earth's surface — or more than the combined land of China and south-east Asia. In the US, more than one billion acres of agricultural land is lying fallow.[7]

There is clearly human demand for food, but because the hungry are also poor, they cannot buy the food they need. Solve the problem of poverty and, in all likelihood, the agricultural efficiency and the food supply will follow. Eating up your greens or not throwing food away because it is past its 'best before' date is not going to help the poor in Africa or Asia.

What Stuart's book does show, however, is just how much slack there is within our food production system and how unnecessarily gloomy is the idea that we cannot feed

---

[7] Food price rises: are biofuels to blame? *spiked*, 7 July 2008

the world. We could already feed the world well just by removing some of the waste in the food chain.

Reducing the environmental impact of food production can really only be tackled in much the same way as reducing other environmental problems, most notably through an abundant supply of cheap, clean energy. Instead of moralising about the wasteful ways of Western consumers, or fretting about how much meat we eat, we'd do far better to look at ways of making global food production more efficient.

Chapter Eight

The wacky world of organic food

It's a lifestyle choice that people can make. There isn't any conclusive evidence either way. It's only four per cent of total farm produce, not 40 per cent and I don't want to say that 96 per cent of our farm produce is inferior because it's not organic.

UK environment minister David Miliband, January 2007

Miliband's statement drew predictable outrage. 'It is not just a lifestyle choice', insisted Soil Association spokesman Robin Maynard. 'In terms of the environment, organic is better. Mr Miliband's own government has recognised in the past that organic food can be better for that. In fact, organic farmers get an extra payment due to this.'[1]

Miliband's remarks were surprising because the superiority of organic food has been taken for granted in recent years. It is assumed that organic food is more 'natural' and therefore by definition healthier and better for the environment—an assumption backed up by government subsidies for inefficient organic farmers. But is this claim true?

Champions of organic food claim that pesticides and other chemicals used in conventional farming have the potential to cause ill-health, either through immediately poisoning us or through causing cancer in the long term. Take this statement from the Soil Association:

[1] Organic farmers hit back at Miliband's food verdict, *Independent*, 8 January 2007

> Chemicals designed to kill: Along with chemical weapons, chemicals used in farming are the only substances that are deliberately released into the environment designed to kill living things. They pose unique hazards to human health and the environment.

Elsewhere on the Soil Association's website we read:

> Around 31,000 tonnes of chemicals are used in farming in the UK each year to kill weeds, insects and other pests that attack crops. There is surprisingly little control over how these chemicals are used in the non-organic sector and in what quantities or combinations. What we do know is that 150 of the available 350 pesticides commonly used have been identified as potentially causing cancer and many of us would have been exposed to these pesticides before we were born.[2]

However, most of our food does not contain residues of these chemicals. Alex Avery, a US critic of organic food, provides some perspective:

> [T]he pesticide residue data are a testament to our technical prowess in detecting incredibly tiny traces of specific chemicals in foods. Note that the synthetic pesticide residues... are consumed in microgram quantities, or one-millionth of a gram.[3]

Given that we tend to buy fruit and veg by the kilo, he notes: 'Remember, this is equivalent to one penny in $10 million, or one inch in 16,000 miles!'

A host of different chemicals can cause cancer in rodents when researchers feed them to the animals in very large quantities. But the minute quantities involved in pesticide residues mean the same chemicals are harmless in food. There is no evidence of anybody ever dying or falling seriously ill from eating food carrying traces of man-made pesticides.

The over-reaction to the dangers from man-made pesticides is in sharp contrast to the complete ignorance shown towards naturally-occurring poisons. Everyday foods are full of natural pesticides. That's hardly a surprise, since we

[2]　Pesticides in your food, Soil Association policy document, 11 August 2006

[3]　Avery, A. (2006) *The Truth About Organic Foods*

tend to choose as crops things that seem resistant to pests and disease. The world-famous biochemist Bruce Ames and his colleague Lois Swirsky Gold make the point clear: 'The natural chemicals that are known rodent carcinogens in a single cup of coffee are about equal in weight to a year's worth of ingested synthetic pesticide residues that are rodent carcinogens.'[4] They are not arguing that coffee is dangerous – far from it. Rather, Ames and Gold are pointing out that the tiny risk from man-made chemicals is actually smaller than other small risks we accept as a normal part of life.

As it happens, as Avery points out, organic produce is not entirely free from chemicals – it is simply that a much narrower range of such chemicals is allowed for food to qualify as 'organic', and such chemicals tend to be used less frequently. Given that some of the things that pesticides are designed to eliminate – like poisonous fungal growths – are pretty dangerous, avoiding their use is not necessarily a good thing. Moreover, the chemicals that are permitted in organic farming are pretty crude weapons like copper and sulphur. Years of research goes into finding pesticides that can kill pests using small quantities while also being harmless to humans. Yet these are rejected by organic farming rules in favour of other substances that are less effective and are much more likely to harm people if not used properly.

That does not mean that organic food is unsafe. What it simply shows is that the advocates of organic farming have some dubious double standards.

Another assertion often made about organic food is that it is more nutritious. It is not clear, in principle, why this might be. However, some studies suggest it might be the case. Avery looks at these studies in detail and finds many of them deeply flawed. One of the best reviews of the evidence, a paper by Woese et al. in 1997, concludes that it is very difficult to conclude anything at all. 'Conventional'

------

[4]   Ames, B., Gold, L. (2003) 'Cancer Prevention and the Environmental Chemical Distraction' in Gough, M. (ed) *Politicizing Science: the Alchemy of Policymaking*

hardly surprising given their greater use in conventional
agriculture. But overall, the authors note:

> With regard to all other desirable nutritional values, it was
> either the case that no major differences were observed in
> physico-chemical analyses between the products from
> different production forms, or contradictory findings did
> not permit any clear statements.[5]

Perhaps organic food simply tastes better. However, in
2011, the consumer organisation *Which?* reported that a trial
it had conducted on tomatoes, broccoli and potatoes found
little difference between organic and conventionally grown
food in terms of nutrition and flavour — and if anything, the
conventionally grown food performed better.

Not only do better quality studies in peer-reviewed jour-
nals show no consistent difference between the two types of
food but, as Avery notes, even some organic advocates
admit this fact. As William Lockeretz of Tufts University
told an organic food conference in 1997:

> I wish I could tell you that there is a clear, consistent nutri-
> tional difference between organic and conventional foods.
> Even better, I wish I could tell you that the difference is in
> favour of organic. Unfortunately, though, from my reading
> of the scientific literature, I do not believe such a claim can
> be responsibly made.

Even if there were nutritional differences between organic
and conventional food, any benefit one way or the other is
likely to be much smaller than the variation caused by other
factors: the variety of a crop used, the other growing conditions, freshness, cooking method. The nutrition we obtain
from a particular food can even be influenced by the foods
we eat with it. Compared with all those factors, any difference between organic and conventional foods is, in practical
terms, irrelevant.

---

[5]   Woese K., D. Lange, C. Boess & K. Werner Böel (1997). 'A comparison
       of organically and conventionally grown foods: results of a review of
       the relevant literature'. *Journal of the Science of Food and Agriculture* 74:
       281–293

Environmental concerns

The environmental case for organic mainly rests upon the pollution caused by producing agricultural chemicals and cleaning up after them. It is certainly true that producing fertilisers, in particular, uses energy and this inevitably means fossil fuels. But the production of chemicals is only one part of the energy used in putting food on our plates. As noted in the previous chapter, many of the assumptions made about what is the most 'green' way to supply food are simply wrong. Big supermarkets and big farmers, with highly efficient logistics, are arguably 'greener' than trying to feed the nation through local farmers' markets and small-scale agriculture.

To maintain the same overall level of food production using organic methods today would require far more land to be used for farming. In developed countries such as the UK, where the efficiency of industrial farming methods has left many small farms redundant, there might be space to indulge a small, land-hungry organic sector. But if we truly pursued the idea of an organic-only economy, the effect on land usage would be dramatic. At a time when environmentalists complain about how wildernesses are being cleared to produce food, the need to clear more land is organic farming's dirty little secret.

It's not merely that a field full of a crop grown by organic methods will be less productive than one employing conventional techniques. There is also the problem of where the organic fertiliser will come from: traditionally, animal manure or plants that capture nitrogen from the air. Either way, land must be taken up in fertiliser production that cannot be used for growing crops.

The other alternative is to grow less food. There is no way, using organic methods, that the world's current population could be sustained on the 37 per cent of land currently used in agriculture. The solution for some, it would appear, is not more food but fewer people. In the words of one organic farmer quoted by Avery, 'I want to argue that production is not the problem. The problem is the imbalance of humans relative to the millions of other species with whom we co-evolved'.

This gets to the nub of the current preoccupation with organic food. The underlying temper of our times is that anything processed or industrialised can be seen as adulterated and harmful, while anything that appears to be natural or close to nature can be regarded as pure and uncorrupted. At issue is the presumed problem with humanity messing with nature. Against this modern prejudice, the precise facts about residues, nutrition or environmental impact are brushed aside.

The 'don't mess with nature' approach is illustrated by the organic movement's attitude to genetic modification. Rather than embracing GM as opening up the possibility of greater control over the properties of plants, with the potential to use fewer chemicals, it is rejected as dangerous interference in nature, ushering in all sorts of unknown potential problems. GM crops have the potential to allow greater productivity, reduced use of pesticides and increased nutrition. Yet the organic movement refuses to engage with the positive potential of GM, preferring to dismiss it all as the work of malevolent agribusiness trying to create monopolies. Of course, producers of GM seeds want to make a profit. But so do the peddlers of over-priced, over-claimed-for organic food.

The roots of organic

The rise of organic food has little to do with a cold assessment of its merits. Rather, the organic movement began largely as a rejection of industrial society and materialism — one that continues today. As an editorial in the *Independent* noted, criticising David Miliband's comments: 'The organic movement is flourishing because it is in tune with the *zeitgeist*, which favours the small and the local and hankers for alternatives to industrial-scale farming and what is an over-cosy relationship between big producers and supermarkets'.[6] It is this suspicion of modern production methods,

---

[6]   Leading article: a matter of choice, *Independent*, 8 January 2007

despite all the benefits they have brought, mixed with over-blown health fears and tied closely to environmentalism, that has allowed organic ideas to become popular.

While the organic movement is often thought of as beginning with Rachel Carson's 1962 book *Silent Spring*, which claimed that pesticides were killing off America's birdlife, the reaction to an agriculture based on man-made chemicals has existed almost as long as have artificial fertilisers. In his book *The Origins of the Organic Movement*, Philip Conford highlights the 1920s, and 1926 in particular, as the moment the organic movement really began.[7] During that year, the Chandos Group of predominantly Anglican thinkers first met in London in the wake of the failed General Strike. Conford argues that this group, who published the *New English Weekly*, were a driving force in popularising organic ideas, some 20 years before the formation of the Soil Association.

A number of other writers emerged in the 1920s promoting broadly similar ideas. Perhaps the most well-known, more for the schools he created than his ideas on agriculture, was Rudolf Steiner. His notion of 'biodynamic' farming sounds downright wacky today, and Avery takes great pleasure in quoting Steiner at length:

> Have you ever thought why cows have horns, or why certain animals have antlers?... The cow has horns in order to send into itself the astral-ethereal formative powers, which, pressing inward, are meant to penetrate right into the digestive organism... Thus in the horn you have something well adapted by its inherent nature to ray back the living and astral properties into the inner life.

So, horns and antlers are like nature's satellite dish for cosmic forces. These forces are concentrated in the digestive system, according to Steiner, which explains the importance of manure:

> What is farm-yard-manure?... [I]t has been inside the organism and has thus been permeated with an astral and ethereal content. In the dung, therefore, we have before us

[7]   Conford, P. (2001), *The Origins of the Organic Movement*

> something ethereal and astral. For this reason it has a
> life-giving and also astralising influence upon the soil.

If you want to improve the fertility of soil, according to
Steiner, you just need to get more 'living forces' into it by the
simple method of filling a horn with manure and burying it
in a field:

> You see, by burying the horn with its filling of manure, we
> preserve in the horn the forces it was accustomed to exert
> within the cow itself... all the radiations that tend to
> etherealize and astralise are poured into the inner hollow
> of the horn.

Steiner sounds like a first-class space cadet. However,
Avery notes that he has a surprising number of followers
even today in the 'biodynamic' movement. For some
reason, biodynamic wines are particularly popular. Then
again, Steiner's ideas are no more scientifically implausible
than those of homeopathy where distilled water, somehow
imprinted with the 'memory' of some active ingredient
long since diluted out of it, can apparently cure all sorts of
ailments.

However, while Steiner certainly had followers, his
presentation was too esoteric for most. A more influential
figure in the long term was Sir Albert Howard. He worked
as an agricultural adviser in India in the 1920s but quickly
concluded that he could learn more from the Indians than
he could teach. He was impressed by the strapping good
health of many of the tribes, particularly the Hunza, and
concluded their rude fitness must be the product of their
food and, by extension, their agriculture.

Central to the ideas that Howard was to promote in later
years was the importance of compost. The Rule of Return —
the idea that vital material from the soil must be returned
through compost and manure — is a key tenet of the organic
movement. Howard advised and supervised the introduction of his Indore system of composting in many places both
in the UK and America. His comments on the ruination of
soil by modern methods could have been made by any
modern environmentalist:

In allowing science to be used to wring the last ounce from
the soil by new varieties of crops, cheaper and more stimulating manures, deeper and more thorough cultivating
machines, hens which lay themselves to death, and cows
which perish in an ocean of milk, something more than a
want of judgment on the part of the organisation is
involved. Agricultural research has been misused to make
the farmer, not a better producer of food, but a more expert
bandit... All goes well as long as the soil can be made to
yield a crop. But soil fertility does not last forever; eventually the land is worn out; real farming dies.[8]

Howard's predictions must have seemed prescient when
American agriculture was doing its best to self-destruct
during the years of the Dust Bowl, when a combination of
inappropriate farming techniques, drought and depression
created the conditions for strong winds to strip vast areas of
topsoil. It is also the case that most farmers use manure and
compost as means of improving soil quality. But Howard
was ultimately wrong.

Better understanding of the use of man-made fertilisers,
selective breeding, and other techniques have greatly
improved crop yields over the past few decades. For example, the Nobel Prize-winning agronomist Norman Borlaug
cross-bred a highly productive but poor quality Japanese
dwarf variety of wheat to produce remarkable leaps in
productivity in the 1960s. Mexican wheat production per
hectare leapt from 1,400 kilogrammes in 1960 to 2,700
kilogrammes in 1963. He repeated the trick in India and
Pakistan; his new seeds helped Indian wheat production
jump from 12 million tonnes in 1965 to 17 million tonnes in
1967 and helped to solve the problem of growing enough
food to feed a rapidly rising population.

What is striking about the early organic pioneers is their
rejection of the modern world. In a world staggering out of
one World War and towards another, via economic and
social turmoil, there were plenty of people who rejected
capitalism. However, most in the organic movement
rejected the communist and socialist alternatives, too, and

---

[8]   Howard, A. (1940), *An Agricultural Testament* quoted in Avery (2006)

recoiled from the class conflict embodied in the General Strike of 1926. The social makeup of those prominent in the early organic movement suggests a group of people being squeezed out of modern society: disillusioned colonials from a declining and increasingly discredited empire, aristocrats seeking to preserve rural life as agricultural workers were replaced by machines, and churchmen trying to find a new setting for religious ideas.

So why are organic ideas that were based on disillusionment with modernity back in fashion today? One explanation could be that economically and politically, Western societies have stagnated over the past 30 years or so, especially in comparison to rapidly developing countries like China, India and the 'Asian tiger' economies. The idea that tomorrow will look radically different from — and better than — today seems unrealistic to many.

Both the political left and right are exhausted, their visions of the future bankrupt. Against this background those who hanker after an imaginary idyllic past, or are fearful of future change, can often exercise disproportionate influence over politics and culture. Alongside the aristocrats like Prince Charles we now have the disillusioned stockbrokers who give up the rat race to sell organic jam, the New Age religionists, and the middle-class hypochondriacs.

Yet history tells us that modern society has made incredible strides in improving living standards, enhancing health and longevity, and developing the global bank of knowledge, through the application of science, industry and reason. And for all the imperfections of the modern world, such gains continue to be made in the developed and developing world alike. Why on earth would we now reject these gains? Growing food more inefficiently, with no nutritional, environmental or aesthetic benefits — as the advocates of organic food would have us do — cannot possibly be a good idea.

Chapter Nine

An alternative to food fears

I began this book with a question: why is it that just when most of the world has solved the problem of finding enough to eat — one of the defining questions of human history — we seem to be more fearful about food than ever before? Even in Britain, once the most important industrialised country in the world, there are plenty of people who can remember when large sections of the population were undernourished. Now the supermarket shelves groan under the weight of affordable, nutritious food, and only the very poorest in British society struggle to get enough good quality food to eat.

While there are still problems associated with food, as there are with almost every aspect of life, these are often exaggerated to an extraordinary degree. For example, we are perfectly capable of growing enough food to feed everyone in the world. That people still go hungry is a problem of politics and economics, not a fundamental natural law. Obesity may make life harder for the small proportion of people who are very overweight, but the idea that great swathes of the population will face serious health problems simply because they are a little fatter than the government deems acceptable is nonsense. The claim that the current generation of children will have shorter lives than their parents is unnecessarily pessimistic, too. School dinners may not be *haute cuisine* but they are not killing our children, and nor are they making them stupid.

The modern food system involves the use of a lot of energy, most of it from fossil fuels. But our eating habits are not wrecking the planet and the alternatives offered to our current food system — like organic food or 'local' production — are a step backwards that are less efficient, will waste land and offer less security of supply. Food panics like those around 'mad cow' disease, genetically modified foods and saturated fat have been an enormous and unnecessary waste of time, resources and money while pointlessly generating anxiety.

So how did we get here? In my view, our societal eating disorder is a product of a range of different factors. Some of these are specific to food, but most are not.

The changing face of food

There have been major changes to the way we produce, purchase and consume food over the past 100 years or so. According to the Office for National Statistics, over the course of the twentieth century, agriculture's share of the UK workforce fell from 11 per cent to two per cent. Yet cereal production leapt from around five million tonnes per year to around 20 million tonnes, even though the area under cultivation is about the same. That's because yields per hectare have shot up, from two tonnes per hectare in 1900 to about eight tonnes per hectare today. What's not to like about such a staggering increase in productivity?

That increase in productivity has been built upon a number of different factors, but the most important are the use of artificial fertilisers, the creation of better crop varieties, and the use of machinery. Thanks to better transportation and storage, less of this crop needs to be wasted.

Technology has also made recent advances in food through the use of genetic modification. Reports in February 2011 suggested that 15 million farmers worldwide are now growing GM crops or one sort or another. GM soya — a staple food in meat production — has become the dominant form, to the extent that British farmers are finding it ever harder to find sufficient non-GM soya to feed animals.

While Europe wrings its hands at the thought of GM foods, and still heavily restricts them, many other countries around the world are embracing GM as an important tool to increase food production.

How we purchase food has changed, too. Once upon a time, women – it was almost invariably women – would need to shop almost every day at a variety of different stores in order to get food for their families. The daily demand was driven by the inability to store food for very long in the absence of refrigeration. Food was fresh, but there was little alternative to fresh food. While this might seem idyllic to some middle-class foodies, the reality was a daily chore for women. The rise of the supermarkets, built particularly on the availability of the fridge and freezer and the motor car (and latterly, the internet), has taken that burden away. Shopping is now a weekly hassle for an hour or so, generally conducted at one of five major supermarket chains that control about 85 per cent of the UK food market. If growing food has been industrialised, so has selling it.

Finally, our consumption habits have changed dramatically. Once, the majority of food was cooked at home, apart from trips to the fish and chip shop; now, eating out is much more common. When I was a lad, eating out meant a trip to a Berni Inn on a special occasion. Now, for most families, eating out in one form or another is routine. Nor is the retreat from the kitchen confined to Britain and America: the second biggest market for McDonald's in the world is, apparently, that bastion of culinary excellence and snobbery, France. Eating in has changed, too, thanks to the ready meal and the takeaway. Why chop up ingredients and sweat over a hot stove when dinner can be provided from a tray – warmed for a few minutes in the oven or the microwave – or delivered by a man on a moped?

This increasing gap between fork and fork – between the one in the soil and the one on the plate – creates many opportunities for food fears to breed, particularly when related to health. From the use of pesticides in the field to additives in our ready meals, from the plastic wrapping in the supermarket to microwaves in our kitchens, there are seemingly endless points in growing, processing and sale of food that are or have been the basis for anxiety.

A retreat from the modern world

Yet these are merely the preconditions for food fears. They do not explain the wide range of negative reactions to food in recent years. After all, we could be — indeed, should be — rejoicing at many of these developments. What a relief for those who live in developed societies to be freed from the grind of producing our own food! What a benefit that this food is produced so cheaply, too, and delivered to us in a way that is so convenient. In a different, more confident era, we would be having street parties to celebrate these achievements, not fretting about how the next mouthful could finish us off.

Our downbeat, backward-looking perspective is also reflected in the solutions that are offered to our current, apparent food problems. Earlier, I mentioned Michael Pollan's recommendation for how to eat better, from his book *In Defence of Food*: 'Eat food. Not too much. Mostly plants.' Both motto and book turn on what he means by 'food': something your great-great grandmother would recognise as food. For Pollan, the weird and wonderful attempts to find new ways to create and deliver food are out of bounds. Food should be home-cooked from fresh ingredients, not provided ready-to-eat by Wal-Mart. But while we could do with being a little more demanding about the quality of what fast-food joints and convenience-food suppliers offer us, Pollan's views are far too conservative, a rejection of the modern as inevitably bad.

Another symptom of this retreat from modern food is the rising number of people growing their own food. In 2008, the Local Government Association called on councils to release more land for allotments because there was a waiting list of 100,000 people who wanted one, though the surge in demand was as much a result of the economic recession as driven by concerns about food safety or the environment.

Having escaped the drudgery of agricultural toil, a sizeable minority of people seem keen to return to it.

To understand what is driving these food fears, we first need to take a step back from food itself to observe that we live in a society that is prone to panicking about all sorts of things.

A fearful society

For a few years, I wrote a column for *spiked* about the scares that regularly cropped up in the media, under the title 'Don't Panic'. While many of these stories were about how a particular kind of food would cause cancer or heart disease, there were plenty of purported threats to us from non-food sources, too: blood clots from sitting still for too long on planes or even in the office; climate change; binge boozing; passive smoking; wifi and mobile phones; how pension liabilities would bankrupt the country.

Past panics have included the 'millennium bug' that was supposedly going to take down the world's most important computer systems when midnight struck on 1 January 2000. The measles, mumps and rubella (MMR) vaccine has been wrongly implicated as a cause of autism in the UK, while a similar and equally baseless vaccine panic in America has focused on the use of a mercury-based preservative called thimoresal. Panics about child sex abuse have led to draconian laws, despite the fact that the threat from strangers is a remote one. And there is the ever-present panic about terrorism, which receives enormous coverage but in reality represents a tiny risk to us.

Looked at this way, fear seems to exist as a social force in its own right, quite separate from any particular cause. Moreover, the things we seem particularly afraid are those threats created by mankind. For example, the accident at the Chernobyl nuclear power plant in 1986 still has an enormous impact on our attitudes to producing energy. The nearest thing to an official death toll from the accident, produced in 2006, suggested that apart from a few dozen people at the scene in the immediate aftermath who received large doses of radiation, the doses of radiation received by those living in the region around the plant have probably caused a very small increase in the risk of cancer. The report suggests 9,000 extra deaths in a population of millions over the course of decades; far, far fewer than are sickened by cigarettes or alcohol. For some commentators on the dangers of radiation, even this small increase in risk as a result of Chernobyl is a gross exaggeration.[1]

Natural disasters, like the Asian tsunami of 2004, have killed many more people than that in a matter of minutes. Yet Chernobyl has almost certainly had a wider impact on people's consciousness — in Europe and America, at least — than any earthquake or flood. This disjuncture between fears created by manmade causes and the reality of natural disaster was brought into sharp relief by events in Japan in 2011 following a massive earthquake and devastating tsunami. While the death toll from the natural disaster ran into many thousands of people, radiation leaks from a nuclear reactor at Fukushima killed no one. Yet it was the overhyped risk of meltdown at the nuclear power plant that dominated the news, at least in the West.

One explanation that has been put forward is that we now know more about the world and have greater control over it. We are simply more aware of the threats that we create. For example, it would be impossible to be scared of pesticide residues on food if we didn't have the sophisticated technology to measure them at the parts-per-billion levels they are found. There's also the fear that one mistake can have a much greater impact because of the scale on which we do things today. So, for example, contamination of food at a processing factory could lead to thousands of people being made ill simultaneously. If greenhouse gas emissions are causing the world to get warmer, that could be bad news for the whole of humanity.

While these things may be true, they don't really explain what is happening because our fears are built on a heightened sense of individual vulnerability. Even societal threats

[1]   See, for example, Allison, W. (2009) *Radiation and Reason*

are ultimately regarded today in terms of how they are a threat to the individual. In his discussion of the contemporary 'culture of fear', sociologist Frank Furedi explains how a sense of vulnerability has been internalised so much that it is now regarded as a 'natural state'.[2]

In this context, problems are all too easily experienced as confirmation of disaster rather than solvable. The wider experience — that living standards and life expectancies generally continue to rise, if a little more slowly than in the past — is ignored in favour of a predisposition towards assuming the worst. The fact that our children, for example, are a little fatter on average than in the past should not be a great concern. But transformed into 'the obesity timebomb', this trend is becomes a deadly threat that is always just over the horizon.

It would be easy to blame the media for this. Newspapers, television and the internet have, to some extent, filled the vacuum where a connection with a close-knit society would have existed. We rely on the media far more than in the past as a way of forming our view about the world — and panics sell papers. But if a fearful view of the world jarred with people's experiences, they would stop reading or change channels. As it is, media gloom-mongering is seen as confirmation of the myriad threats to our bodies and selves; and the more directly the reported threats relate to us — as in the food we eat — the more quickly the panics are ingested.

The rise of the fearmongers

But while the media have played a small part in promoting the culture of fear, other social actors have been more important. As the sociologist David Altheide has argued, 'fear does not just happen; it is socially constructed and then manipulated by those who seek to benefit'.[3] Numerous individuals and groups — Frank Furedi refers to them as

---

[2]   Furedi, F. (1997) *Culture of Fear*
[3]   Altheide, D.L. (2002) *Creating Fear; News and the Construction of Crisis*, quoted in The only thing we have to fear is the 'culture of fear' itself, *spiked*, 4 April 2007

'fear entrepreneurs' — have actively stoked up food panics
in order to promote their own policy agendas; Jamie Oliver
is a good example of someone who has taken a mish-mash
of relatively small problems — like obesity and classroom
discipline — mixed them together and heated them up in the
name of promoting his ideas about how we should be fed. In
the eyes of campaigners, everything is an 'epidemic', a
'plague' or a 'timebomb'.

Food campaigns in particular seem to be overwhelmingly informed by a middle-class outlook. The experts here
are celebrity chefs — the culinary equivalent of taxi drivers;
the loudest voices seem to be those who think it is their place
to tell the masses how to live their lives. And unfortunately,
we have been rather timid in telling these caring experts to
get out of our kitchens. One heartwarming exception was in
2008, when Jamie Oliver tried to persuade the fans of
Rotherham United to take advantage of his cookery lessons
in the town. He was greeted with a rousing chorus of 'Who
ate all the pies?'

Food campaigners would have limited influence, were it
not for their disproportionate impact in the political domain
in recent years. Having given up on real politics, designed
to change the world, Western governments have been
pro-active in promoting 'the politics of behaviour', pushing
policy agendas that attempt to micromanage people's
lives — often in the name of 'public health'. As a strategy for
connecting with a largely disengaged electorate, it works, at
least to the extent that once the populace is convinced that
'something must be done' about an issue, then the government can step forward to fulfill that role.

So after Jamie Oliver's school meals crusade, the New
Labour government was only too happy to find a few hundred million pounds to fund his ideas. The government
then went further, using food as a means of teaching
children the 'right' ideas about health while disciplining
parents who had the temerity to have non-approved ideas
about what to feed their children.

When the Conservative-Liberal coalition took office in
May 2010, it may have appeared that things would change.

The new health secretary, Andrew Lansley, was critical of Jamie Oliver's approach in comments made to the British Medical Association conference in June 2010. 'If we are constantly lecturing people and trying to tell them what to do, we will actually find that we undermine and are counterproductive in the results that we achieve.'

However, Lansley was still primarily interested in how government could change the unhealthy behaviours of the population.[4] He was just quibbling about the methods. So, by December, Lansley was launching a new phase of the Change4Life campaign to get us all eating less and exercising more while the government was considering the creation of healthy eating guidelines for 'early years' children — those older than babies but too young for primary schools. It seems that under the coalition, no age group can be spared from having its meals watched over by the state. For all the coalition's stated interest in rolling back the 'nanny state', when it comes to food and health issues, it seems prepared to go even further.

The role of government in recent years has been to exacerbate food fears, rather than taking the responsible course of action and calming things down. For example, having attempted (quite correctly) to allay fears about BSE — 'mad cow' disease — the decision to ban beef on the bone in 2002 on the basis of theoretical risks about the transmission of an infectious agent was both disproportionate and undermined the idea that government could be trusted when it suggested that food was safe. Now, precaution and overreaction seem to be the order of the day.

A good example of this precautionary, fear-inducing approach was the reaction to the risk from a red dye, Sudan-I, in 2005. Some chilli powder from India had been adulterated with a dye to make it look redder. The quantity of dye involved would have been small. However, nobody in the UK consumed the chilli powder directly. Instead, it was used as an ingredient in Worcestershire sauce, thus

---

[4]   Minister rejects 'Jamie Oliver approach' on health, BBC News, 30 June 2010

diluting its effect further. But nobody consumed the sauce directly, either. It was added to a variety of ready meals, reducing the quantities of dye that people would have been exposed to down to absolutely tiny levels. Even then, the dye would only have been potentially carcinogenic in quantities far greater than would ever actually be eaten — and the particular chemical in the dye that was apparently a threat also occurs naturally in carrots. Nonetheless, 350 processed foods had to be withdrawn from supermarket shelves. It seems that governments would prefer that we believe everything possible is being done rather than take a cool look at the real dangers involved in any particular situation.[5]

The antidote to our eating disorder

The aim of this book has been to try to bring a semblance of balance to the food debate. At present, any discussion of food seems to assume that we are screwing up the planet or signing our own death warrants every time we tuck in to anything that isn't organic and produced by someone we're on first-name terms with. I personally find the vision of food promoted by foodie magazines and Channel 4 campaign shows to be rather unappetising.

We could try treating our collective eating disorder, first, with a generous serving of scepticism. Such scepticism is often one-sidedly applied to big business, which, it is argued, is only there to sell poor-quality, over-priced food without regard to the costs to our health or the planet. While it would be naive to think that multinational corporations are in business to feed the world, rather than turn a profit, it is in our own interests to take a balanced view of the effect of supermarkets, food processors and agri-business. If we do, we will find that they provided, on balance, a considerable net benefit to society even if there is also room for criticism of what they do.

---

[5]   See 'The dangers of dye', *spiked*, 21 February 2005
http://bit.ly/gLN5BY

In turn, scepticism needs to be applied to campaigners and governments who spend time attempting to scare us into following one policy or another. What is the truth about the threats we are told we face, like obesity, pesticides or climate change? Do these campaigners really have our interests at heart?

The other thing we need is a little historical perspective. The absence of alternative ways of seeing society's future seems also to have crushed our ability to comprehend the past. But when we do take a look back, we can see how far we've come, how much better off we are now than in the past. Suddenly, today's problems seem small by comparison. And the gains of the past should give us great confidence about humanity's capacity to cope with the trials and tribulations of the future.

Another remedy for our eating disorder could lie in greater trust — not of the campaigners whom we seem to trust rather too much, but in our own experiences and the standards of the modern world. After all, why aren't we afraid of absolutely everything? When I go to a supermarket to buy food from strangers, that was grown, transported, cooked and packaged by strangers, they could have done all sorts of things to it. How do I know that it will be safe to eat?

There are plenty of reasons to be confident. Firstly, I know that there are rules imposed on every part of the food chain to ensure high standards (sometimes to a ludicrous degree). Secondly, I know from my own personal experience, and from the people I know, that the food has been safe before. Thirdly, I know that a big supermarket chain has a material interest in maintaining a good reputation. So there's a powerful mixture of trust and accountability here that makes buying food reassuringly predictable.

This panic on a plate will not disappear overnight; it is too bound up with lots of other social changes for that. But a generous serving of scepticism, with a large side order of faith in the people around us, would allow us to enjoy our food in peace.

Afterword

The German E. coli outbreak

The main text for *Panic on a Plate* was completed in April 2011. Within a few weeks, however, a new event unfolded that confirmed some of the themes discussed in the book: a deadly outbreak of food poisoning in northern Germany.

The first cases of Enterohaemorrhagic *E. coli* (EHEC) occurred around 2 May. However, the seriousness of the situation became clear with an announcement by the German health authorities on 24 May that there had been 80 cases and three deaths from haemolytic uraemic syndrome (HUS) — a condition that damages the kidneys — caused by EHEC. On 25 May, the authorities suggested there may be a link with raw salad vegetables and advised consumers to avoid them.

By the following day, it looked like a culprit had been found: Hamburg Institute for Hygiene and the Environment (HU) said that three of four cucumbers found to be positive for *E. coli* had came from Spain. 'The HU has clearly identified a cucumber from Spain as a carrier of *E. coli*', declared the German health ministry. The result, however, was not a solution to the crisis but an almighty diplomatic row between Spain and Germany, with the Spanish protesting that there was no proof that their produce was to blame. Russia, not content to wait for confirmation, banned imports of vegetables from Germany and Spain within days.

By 31 May, however, it was clear that pinning the blame on Spanish cucumbers had been premature. The *E. coli* strain found on them was different to the deadly new variety. Cornelia Prüfer-Storcks, Hamburg's state health minister, who had been the first to announce a possible link, explained: 'It would have been irresponsible to withhold a well-founded suspicion given the high number of illnesses. Protecting life is more important than protecting financial interests.' Nonetheless, Spanish farmers were demanding compensation for millions of euros of lost sales. With no explanation for the outbreak in sight, Russia banned imports of all fresh vegetables from all 27 EU members states on 2 June, despite the fact that all the cases of EHEC poisoning had been among people who either lived in or had visited northern Germany.

It took until 5 June before the immediate villain of the piece really became clear: bean sprouts. Circumstantial evidence had built up that a high proportion of those infected had eaten bean sprouts from an organic farm south of Hamburg. Although bacteriological tests failed to confirm the link, those who ate bean sprouts from the nursery were almost nine times more likely to have been made ill than those who had not.

However, other complications have since arisen. Later in June, other batches of cases appeared in France and Sweden.

The ultimate cause of the outbreak is harder to identify. In the case of France, an initial theory was that a British seed company had supplied infected seeds, though this was vigorously denied. On 30 June, the European Centre for Disease Prevention and Control (ECDC) suggested that fenugreek seeds imported in 2009 and 2010 from Egypt might be to blame, but that there was 'much uncertainty'. That didn't stop the EU from banning imports of *all* seeds and beans from Egypt a few days later.

The latest figures at the time of writing are that 16 countries in Europe and North America have reported 3,941 cases of EHEC infection—3,804 of them in Germany—including 52 fatalities. But it isn't just the immediate deaths that are a concern. Many of those who have suffered from HUS have also suffered permanent kidney damage and will need either dialysis or kidney transplants to survive.

This has been a serious outbreak, but a little perspective is required, too. Here are some lessons we can usefully draw from the EHEC outbreak.

Lesson one:
This is still a relatively small problem

Whenever a new disease appears, the uncertainty about what it is, where it comes from and how to deal with it can be very disruptive for a period of time. Fairly localised incidents, like this recent one centred on northern Germany, can place a major strain on medical services. But 52 deaths, while tragic for each and every family concerned, are not many in the grand scheme of things, either.

For example, according to EU statistics, in Germany in 2008 there were over 64,000 cases of the most common form of food poisoning, campylobacteriosis, and 876 cases of the kind of toxin-producing *E. coli* infection in the current outbreak (though the particular bacterium involved in the recent outbreak seems to be completely new).

Overall, there are just under 900,000 deaths from all causes in Germany in each year. The number of deaths from EHEC pales in comparison to those from the wide range of causes that we are more familar with, like heart disease, strokes and cancer. The deaths related to EHEC are 'news' partly because they represent something 'new', but also because they seem like the latest confirmation that we are extremely vulnerable, that we're just one slice of misfortune away from disaster. To really understand the *E. coli* scare, therefore, we need to be sensitive to the fact that we live in a society with a very high sensitivity to risk.

As described earlier in *Panic on a Plate*, these fears are not simply about health — although health scares like swine flu, SARS and obesity are very important — but derive from a variety of causes including computer problems (the 'millennium bug'), climate change, terrorism, and many more.

With so many panics flying about, it is clear that the presentiment towards feeling vulnerable and 'at-risk' exists quite separately from any particular problem and tends to greatly magnify the apparent importance of such problems.

Lesson two:
Speculation is dangerous

The early suggestion from German officials, that the cause might be Spanish cucumbers, did not solve anything; the effect was simply to devastate Spanish exports, with Spanish farmers claiming that the incident could cost them €200million per week in lost sales. Now, it is the turn of Egyptian farmers to suffer losses as a result of the blame being pointed at them.

While the outcry for some answers may be difficult to resist, this speculation has been costly and counterproductive. Finding a common source of infection, amongst the wide variety of foods that German consumers had eaten, must have been difficult, but there is simply no shortcut to establishing the facts. Yet, it seems, health officials can't help themselves. How else to explain French finger-pointing at British seeds or the ECDC announcement about Egyptian seeds? Unfortunately, there are rarely any quick routes to understanding how a novel illness has come about.

It would be far better for health officials to offer general advice about food handling and to put risks into perspective than to stoke up fears by such precautionary announcements.

Lesson three:
Anti-technology sentiments make things worse

Some of the major breakthroughs in food safety, like pasteurisation and canning, have come about through applying new technologies to destroying infection. The best, and most common, method of infection control is cooking. Properly cooked food is, with a few exceptions, completely safe to eat. However, that doesn't help when the food in question is served raw.

Yet a method for dealing with this problem has been available for many years: irradiation. Giving food a short blast of gamma rays, electrons or x-rays is enough to kill-off nearly all the bugs within it. This is not only an excellent protection from pathogens, but it also enables food to stay fresh for longer; for example, irradiated strawberries stay fresh for weeks rather than days. (So, not only safer food but, in theory, less food waste, too.) While irradiation is not suitable for every foodstuff, and is best applied in conjunction with other food-hygiene measures, it would be a good solution for cucumbers and bean sprouts, for example.

Yet the EU as a whole only approves irradiation for one kind of food: spices. The technology is used in a number of member states, like the Netherlands and France, for a wider group of foods including poultry and frog's legs. Ironically, it appears that it was Germany that blocked wider EU approval of irradiation. Here's another comparison worth chewing on: the number of proven deaths from the nuclear accident at Chernobyl was about 50. Misguided fears about radiation, which have led to the blocking of irradiation as a food treatment, may just have led to about 50 more deaths.

Lesson four:
Our food system is not 'broken'

Food production is now more efficient than ever before, providing consumers with cheaper, more durable produce at lower prices and with greater convenience.

Yet for many food commentators and campaigners, Big Food is a disaster waiting to happen. So it's no surprise that some leapt on events in Germany to suggest we need to retreat from industrialised food production. In early June, just before the announcement that organic bean sprouts seemed to be the immediate source of the outbreak, food writer Joanna Blythman provided *Daily Mail* readers with a litany of dangers lurking in our salads, from sewage contamination to pesticides, all based on 'ifs' and 'maybes'.

In her *Observer* column a few days later, Blythman was even more sweeping in her condemnation of mass production, declaring that by its very nature, our industrialised, globalised food system begets public-health problems. It is geared to churning out vast volumes of food and raising productivity, but at the lowest cost. So farmers and growers are pushed to make savings by cutting corners and adopting intensive practices, which open up unprecedented risks that are graver all the time: everything from toxins from GM crops turning up in foetal blood, through sickly, cloned calves dying soon after birth, to the creation of more virulent superbugs.

Blythman demanded a 'radically different model of food and agriculture, one that is based on the largely untapped potential of small-scale, much more regional production and food distribution'.

Yet Blythman seemed to contradict herself, noting that the UK's worst *E. coli* outbreak, in 1996 in Scotland — which killed 21 people — originated in a small butcher's shop, not some mega meat-processor. Small is not necessarily beautiful, and 'natural' isn't any safer than 'manmade' or 'processed'. As we develop larger-scale production and distribution methods, appropriate regulations should be in place to ensure good standards of hygiene, but dealing with reams of safety regulations is far easier for large producers who can employ specialist staff to ensure the implementation of such rules. (The key word is 'appropriate'; producers of some tasty traditional products have been hurt by overzealous regulation, too.)

Another claim made is that agricultural use of antibiotics is creating 'superbugs' that cannot be treated. The most famous of these superbugs is MRSA, which kills thousands of people each year in UK hospitals. Whether these superbugs are really a product of agriculture, however, is another matter.

Antibiotics are used in two ways in agriculture. Firstly, for the direct treatment of disease, in a similar way to the use of antibiotics in humans. Secondly, in much smaller quantities, as a way of promoting growth by dampening down the production of certain bacteria in an animal's guts. With the sheer volume of bacteria produced all the time, it is possible that antibiotic-resistant versions may appear. The suggestion is that if these caused disease in humans, then antibiotics may be unable to kill them.

For example, in a column for the *Independent* in June 2011, Johann Hari warns of the dangers of routine antibiotic use in farm animals:

> In the United States, Latin America, and Asia, animals being farmed for meat and milk are being automatically given antibiotics in their food all day—irrespective of whether they are healthy or sick. It's like slathering your child's cornflakes with antibiotics, all year round. Some 80 per cent of all antibiotics in the US go straight into farm animals…. It's like taking bacteria to the gym and giving them a constant work-out—and then unleashing them on the rest of us.

Hari quotes a 1976 study in the *New England Journal of Medicine* as proof that 'our factory farms are massively artificially accelerating' the development of superbugs. Cramming together a whole bunch of disparate concerns, Hari practically splutters into meltdown:

> Small groups of rich people, determined to maximise profits, are buying or bamboozling politicians into serving their interests and into ignoring the interests of the vast majority of the population. This is the trend that is making it so hard to (say) reregulate the banks to prevent another global crash, or prevent the unravelling of the climate.

I hope he had a chance for a nice lie-down after working himself up into such a fevered state.

But while antibiotic-resistant bacteria *can* be produced in such circumstances, that doesn't mean that they will go on to make people sick or that agriculture is the main source of this problem. A study in 2000 attempted to get some measure of what impact animal antibiotic use had on the overall picture of antibiotic resistance. The authors surveyed experts in a variety of different kinds of bacteria, finding that most believed the impact of animal antibiotic use had little effect on antibiotic resistance, particularly in the case of the most important antibiotic-resistant infection in humans, MRSA.

The organisation that funded the study quoted by Hari, the Animal Health Institute in Washington, argues that while antibiotic resistance is possible from the use of antibiotics in animals, 'data from the Centers for Disease Control and Prevention (CDC) show that levels of resistant foodborne bacteria in humans are decreasing. USDA data show that the presence of pathogens on raw meat has been reduced, and the CDC FoodNet has reported a 23 per cent decline in foodborne illness since 1996'. As a World Health Organisation report in 1999 noted, 'It is highly probable that the greatest stimulant to the production of resistant bacteria in humans is the use of antibiotics in human medicine'. In other words, over-prescribing of antibiotics by doctors is a far more important cause of antibiotic resistance than anything done in animals, whether or not any connection is ultimately found between antibiotics and the EHEC outbreak in Germany.

Food is both essential to our existence and a perennial source of illness. We cannot ever hope to completely eliminate food-borne illness, but we can and should learn lessons from serious incidents like the current one in Germany so that we can improve food hygiene in the future. Over-reaction, however, is not helpful. Confronting problems with prejudices — like that the idea that 'natural is best' or that large-scale food production is killing us — won't help, either.

Modern food production is overwhelmingly a success story, something to be celebrated. If that does create some problems along the way, we should find ways to tackle those problems, not retreat to some mythical idyllic past. Indeed, we should be thankful for all the improvements in food safety that industrialised food production has brought. While the small-and-local-and-organic-is-beautiful crowd seems desperate to use tragedies like the deaths in Germany as a stick to beat Big Food with, the fact is that the past they romanticise was much worse than the safe, cheap and plentiful food we enjoy today.

Index